THE
ATKINS
SHOPPING
GUIDE

By Robert C. Atkins, M.D.

Atkins for Life
Dr. Atkins' New Carbohydrate Gram Counter
Dr. Atkins' Age-Defying Diet
Dr. Atkins' Vita-Nutrient Solution
Dr. Atkins' Quick & Easy New Diet Cookbook
Dr. Atkins' New Diet Cookbook
Dr. Atkins' New Diet Revolution
Dr. Atkins' Health Revolution
Dr. Atkins' Nutrition Breakthrough
Dr. Atkins' Nutrition SuperEnergy Diet Cookbook
Dr. Atkins' SuperEnergy Diet
Dr. Atkins' Diet Cookbook
Dr. Atkins' Diet Revolution

Coming Soon in Hardcover
Atkins Diabetes Revolution
by Robert C. Atkins, M.D.

And Don't Miss
The Atkins Essentials
by Atkins Health & Medical Information Services

THE
ATKINS
SHOPPING
GUIDE

 ATKINS HEALTH & MEDICAL INFORMATION SERVICES

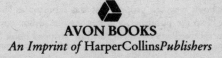

AVON BOOKS

An Imprint of HarperCollinsPublishers

The information presented in this work is in no way intended as medical advice or as a substitute for medical counseling. The information should be used in conjunction with the guidance and care of your physician. Consult your physician before beginning this program as you would with any weight-loss or weight-maintenance program. Your physician should be aware of all medical conditions that you may have as well as the medications and supplements you are taking. Those of you on diuretics or diabetes medications should proceed only under a doctor's supervision. As with any plan, the weight-loss phases of this nutritional plan should not be used by patients on dialysis or by pregnant or nursing women.

All information concerning branded products in this book was taken from product labels in the marketplace or listed on websites at or about the time of publication. Atkins Nutritionals, Inc., is not responsible for updating formulation modifications made after the print date of this book. Atkins Nutritionals is not responsible for any errors or omissions in the printing process.

AVON BOOKS
An Imprint of HarperCollins*Publishers*
10 East 53rd Street
New York, New York 10022-5299

Copyright © 2004 by Atkins Nutritionals, Inc.
ISBN: 0-06-072200-2
www.avonbooks.com

First Avon Books paperback printing: May 2004

Avon Trademark Reg. U.S. Pat. Off. and in Other Countries, Marca Registrada, Hecho en U.S.A.
HarperCollins® is a trademark of HarperCollins Publishers Inc.

Printed in the U.S.A.

10 9 8 7 6 5 4 3 2 1

Acknowledgments

Written by the Atkins Health & Medical Information Services team, this book builds upon the longstanding commitment to providing solid information to make it as easy as possible for people to do Atkins.

Michael Bernstein, senior vice president of Atkins Health & Medical Information Services, manages the group's efforts to continually offer information and educational materials directly to people, with the hope that through understanding the truth about Atkins, more and more people can manage their weight and improve their health. Vice president and editorial director Olivia Bell Buehl oversaw the development of this book. Without executive editor Christine Senft, M.S., a nutritionist, this book would never have seen the light of day. She worked tirelessly with a team of consultants to organize the vast amount of information and present it in a reader-friendly way, all the while ensuring its accuracy. Nutritionist Colette Heimowitz, M.S., vice president and director of education and research, provided overall guidance. Our food scientists, Matt Spolar, vice president of product development, and Paul Bruns, Ph.D., manager of scientific affairs, reviewed the manuscript and provided valuable assistance in translating the often arcane language of food science into terminology normal mortals can understand. Other members of the marketing staff were equally helpful.

Our consultant team, all of whom regularly contribute to *www.atkins.com* and to other Atkins informational publica-

tions, included Martha Schueneman, Janet Blake, Lynn
Prowitt-Smith, Pamela Mitchell and Andrea Israel. They did
the legwork that was essential to getting *The Atkins
Shopping Guide* from concept to the book you hold in your
hands. They trawled the supermarkets and natural foods
stores looking for acceptable and not-so-acceptable products, often alerting us to items we had never heard of, and
wrote up their findings. Martha Schueneman also produced
many of the sidebars that make the book even more helpful.
Finally, this book would not have been possible without the
efforts of assistant Amanda Dorato. A recent graduate of the
Culinary Institute of America, Amanda reviewed the data on
each and every product, a huge task that she took on with
energy and good humor.

The team at Avon Books pulled out all the stops to get this
book done in record time. Editor Sarah Durand suggested
the basic idea for the book, and then applied all her editorial skills to help make it as useful and well organized as possible. Special thanks to Michael Morrison, Libby Jordan,
Darlene DeLillo, Anne Marie Spagnuolo, Elizabeth Glover,
Juliette Shapland, and Jeremy Cesarec.

Contents

Contents

Introduction

The typical supermarket can hold about 50,000 items, and approximately 11,000 new food products are introduced each year, making it possible for you to find just about any food you want—as well as some you didn't even *know* you wanted! But among all this abundance lurks confusion. The sheer number of choices can be overwhelming and enormously time-consuming. And if you are just becoming acquainted with the Atkins Nutritional Approach™ (ANA™), the typical shopping trip can be doubly frustrating. Alas, much of what beckons from the well-stocked shelves is simply inappropriate for doing Atkins. Just a few short years ago, people often felt challenged by the task of finding food products suitable for doing Atkins. Today, the tables have turned, and with the explosion of items labeled "low carb," "controlled carb," "reduced carb," and "no carb," you may find yourself baffled by the many options.

Let's be honest, you shouldn't need a Ph.D. in marketing (or chemistry) to steer your shopping cart through the aisles with skill and exit the store with healthy, delicious foods. But how can you achieve your health and weight-control goals if you're not sure you're buying Atkins-appropriate foods? Clearly, you need to be able to find the foods that help you succeed and avoid those that can sabotage your best intentions. And now that controlling carbs has become so popular, some foods that proclaim themselves low in carbs may not be all that low or may contain ingredients unsuitable for someone doing Atkins. In true Atkins tradition, this book provides people like you with the information needed to make informed decisions.

➤ HOW DID WE WRITE THIS BOOK? ◄

To get in the heads of folks like you, we sent five "real" people from various parts of the country out into the marketplace. All have families. Some are already confirmed Atkins followers; others are beginning to explore the low-carb way of eating. Each visited a number of stores in his or her area: Two members of our research team live in a major city, two in the suburbs and one in a rural area. They went to different types of stores in their hunt for products, carefully scrutinizing the ingredients list and Nutrition Facts panel for each one, then reported their findings.

➤ WHAT IS THIS BOOK ABOUT? ◄

First and foremost the purpose of *The Atkins Shopping Guide* is to help you do Atkins right. It is designed to make it easy for you to fill your fridge and pantry with the appropriate foods. As Atkins followers shared with us their frustrations in finding suitable foods, we grasped the tremendous need for this book by anyone who does Atkins—or is thinking about starting the program. *The Atkins Shopping Guide* puts you in command by teaching you how to be a smart low-carb shopper. Before you even leave your house, this practical companion will introduce you to many of the foods you will find at the store. Or, you can take it along to help you scan the shelves, obtaining just the information you need, at a glance.

We know that many of you like to shop in a variety of stores, from supermarkets, club stores and superstores to natural foods stores. (Some nutrition stores also carry a limited line of food products.) Each type of store has its advantages, from vast selection in supermarkets and superstores, to good value in club stores. Natural foods stores have a great range of low-carb foods and are often staffed by people who are well informed about controlling carbohydrates. So we have organized the book into two major sections: Part 1 covers supermarkets (and applies to the superstores and club stores); Part 2 covers the natural foods (and nutrition) stores.

An important point: This book does not *recommend* foods. The only foods we can vouch for are those that come from Atkins Nutritionals or carry an Atkins endorsement. We have not tasted other manufacturers' products. Nor do we know how the information on their Nutrition Facts panels is computed. We merely list the products we have found on store shelves and report on the nutritional information on manufacturers' labels or websites. However, when a food which initially might appear to be acceptable for doing Atkins has ingredients you might not be aware of or ones that we consider unacceptable, we will point this out so you can make your own decision. But, in essence, it's up to you to use the information provided herein to determine which foods to purchase to stay on track, taking into consideration the phase of Atkins you're in, your individual carbohydrate threshold, and your health goals. While we briefly explain the Atkins Nutritional Approach (see page 21), this book is not a substitute for *The Atkins Essentials* or *Dr. Atkins' New Diet Revolution,* the cornerstone publications for understanding and accurately following the program.

We encourage you to be proactive. Remember, for a store to succeed, it must respond to shoppers' needs—and demands. Once you become aware of food products that support the Atkins lifestyle, you can be part of a potent force to change what turns up on the shelves of the stores you patronize. If you do not see some of the foods you read about in this book in your store, ask the manager to order them. By speaking up, you will help not just yourself but the many others who want more low-carb options.

➤ A NEW FOOD CATEGORY ◄

In the last few years, scientific research has consistently validated the principles upon which Atkins is based. As a result, in the last year we have witnessed a huge growth in the food category pioneered by Atkins Nutritionals: products specifically created for people following a controlled-carb lifestyle. Recently, even major players in the food business have jumped on the low-carb bandwagon. (Yes, the very same companies that have pushed the low-fat dogma for years are now singing a different tune!) In fact, industry analysts predict that we are presently seeing just the tip of the iceberg as more and more people adopt this healthy way of eating. Even if we included every item on store shelves on the day this book goes to press, by the time you buy it, there will be new products in the marketplace that are not found here. It is simply impossible for this book to be 100% comprehensive. (Likewise, not every store will have every item we list.) For that reason, we plan to update it regularly and welcome your contributions. Do let us know when you come across products that you feel should be added by e-mailing us at *shoppingguide@atkins.com*. Be sure to provide the full name of the manufacturer and a website or other contact information.

Controlled-carb products often include as-yet unfamiliar ingredients. In the appropriate sections, we'll tell you about ingredients such as sugar alcohols, resistant starches, and organic acids, which make it possible to create delicious, low-carb foods. As the industry leader, and with the ANA as the only low-carb approach that has been validated by science, Atkins Nutritionals is committed to helping ensure your success on our four-phase program. That's why Atkins products were created to support people in various phases. If an Atkins product is not suitable for Induction—or another phase—the label makes that clear. Packaging also includes the Atkins Net Carb Seal, which indicates the number of grams of Net Carbs, the only carbs you need to count when you do Atkins. (Net Carbs are the only ones that impact blood sugar.) To ensure that you consume controlled-carb products properly, please follow this critical advice:

- Eat them only to support a total controlled-carb dietary approach that brings carbs into the right balance with fish, meat, eggs, and other forms of protein and healthy fats.
- Remember that controlled-carb products are not a substitute for whole foods. Make sure you are eating enough leafy greens and other vegetables before you add controlled-carb foods.
- Eat only products that are suitable for the phase of Atkins you are in.
- Always be guided by your personal carbohydrate threshold for weight loss or weight maintenance. (For more on this, see "Understanding Your Carb Threshold" on page 14.)
- Eat controlled-carb foods in moderation as part of the balanced diet cited above.

Even though Atkins offers a wide array of products that make it easier to do Atkins, we are the first to say that doing Atkins is not about filling up on controlled-carb products. The primary Atkins message is to control your carbs and eat whole foods, which is why we begin with and devote so much space to the perimeter of the supermarket, where whole foods are found.

Nor can you eat a few controlled-carb products but continue to eat a high-carb/high-fat diet and expect to improve your health and control your weight. In fact, the combination of high-fat *and* high-carb foods is a recipe for health problems. Put simply, do Atkins by the book, and then—and only then—use controlled-carb products appropriately to help you achieve optimal health.

Sadly, there are many products out there that do not meet the criteria to which Atkins adheres. Many of these new products are much higher in carbs than is suitable for someone doing Atkins, as you will see in certain product listings.

Because the FDA has not yet specifically defined the use of the term "low carb," different manufacturers use this term loosely. Don't let this fad approach to marketing sway you. Remember Atkins has been making controlled-carb products for years, so you can trust us.

Bottom line, it's great to have many options, but be sure that you are using those products that support your success. You may be able to convince your mind that you are doing Atkins because you are snacking on low-carb chips instead of regular potato chips, but your body will not be fooled.

➤ WHOLE FOODS ◄

While foods specifically developed for individuals who are controlling their carbs have made it easier to do Atkins, there is also a myriad of foods that are naturally low in carb content. And we are not just talking about meat. Atkins is all about controlling carbs—and eating only nutrient-dense carbs—while enjoying a wide variety of protein sources, along with natural fats. The foundation of the ANA is natural, unprocessed foods such as poultry, fish, soy products, cheese, eggs, nuts and seeds, fats such as olive oil and avocado, along with a myriad of carb foods. Initially, carbs take the form of salad greens and other vegetables—and as you proceed through the four phases of the program—you add moderate portions of berries and other fruits, legumes like lentils and chickpeas, starchy vegetables like carrots and sweet potatoes, and even whole grains. As the basis of the ANA and the foods you should eat the most, these foods are sold pretty much the way Mother Nature made them.

➤ NATURALLY LOW IN CARBS ◄

Many other minimally processed foods as diverse as salmon pâté and old-fashioned oatmeal are well suited to doing Atkins. Others, such as salsa, preserves, and yogurt, which are typically sugar-laden, can now be found in lower-carb versions. How can you know which items pass muster and which you should avoid? We'll help you distinguish the nutritious products from those that you should stay away from with a ten-foot pole. For instance, while canned pumpkin puree is fine, beware of canned pumpkin pie mix, which adds sugar and spices to the puree and can wallop your weight-loss efforts with 18 grams of Net Carbs in one-third cup.

➤ HOW IS THIS BOOK ORGANIZED? ◄

Although not all supermarkets or superstores are laid out the same way, most retailers follow certain conventions. For example, the produce, dairy, and meat sections, along with other fresh foods, tend to be located around the perimeter of the store, while sections such as snacks, beverages, canned goods, and baking supplies usually occupy the interior aisles. With this in mind, we have divided the book into two major parts: Part 1 covers the supermarket and is further subdivided into the perimeter and the center aisles. You should be doing most of your shopping on the edges of the store and where most foods are Atkins-friendly for some or all phases. In the thornier arena—the interior aisles of the store—acceptable choices are few and far between and caution is the operative word. Part 2 visits natural foods stores, where specialty items not typically found in supermarkets or superstores are more likely to be stocked. Of course, many supermarkets and superstores now have natural foods or health food sections. More and more supermarkets, superstores, and natural foods stores are also setting up special sections that group many of the products specifically marketed as low carb.

Depending upon where you live, you may be able to find products we have listed in Part 2 in your supermarket.

Likewise, some items listed in Part 1 may be more typically found in a natural foods store in your locality. Space does not allow us to repeat foods in both sections. We have provided cross-references in many places, but you should familiarize yourself with all sections. When it comes to the Atkins line of food products, availability is broadening at lightning speed, and you can find many of them in natural foods stores as well as supermarkets, which is why we have listed them in both sections. When a category includes Atkins-brand foods, we list them first. We've also provided a complete listing of Atkins products at the back of the book.

➤ HOW TO USE THIS BOOK ◄

Within each part, we have organized the content by aisles, such as Condiments or Frozen Foods, and then by categories such as Salad Dressings, Pasta Sauces, Marinades, and the like. Again, whenever possible, we have made cross-references. For example, olives appear in the Deli section, in Canned Foods, and in Condiments. Sausages likewise turn up in the Meat section, in Frozen Foods, and in the Deli section. If you are exploring a whole category of foods, turn to the appropriate aisle and then to the category; to find a particular product, use the index.

➤ A WORLD OF CHOICES ◄

The United States is a true cultural melting pot. To mirror this diversity, we've included numerous ethnic foods and ingredients, which are disbursed throughout the book in appropriate categories. Many of these foods—like guacamole, hummus, and sauerkraut—have become mainstream. However, providing the nutrition information for certain ethnic specialties, like *nam pla* (fish sauce), wasabi paste, chipotle en adobo and chorizo, will no doubt make it easier for many to remain true to family and cultural traditions as they follow a controlled-carb lifestyle. But even if they're not part of *your* ethnic background, be sure to experiment with some of these foods—they may just open your eyes to a whole new world of flavors.

➤ WHAT INFORMATION IS PROVIDED ◄

BRAND NAMES: For much of Part 1, which covers primarily whole, unprocessed foods such as cheese, fresh fish, fruits, and vegetables, brand names are irrelevant. Likewise, for categories that do not offer significant differences among brands—hot sauce, mustard, cream, and bottled capers, for example—we provide general guidelines, rather than list individual brands. Instead, we confine our use of brand names to situations in which you could not readily select the wheat from the chaff without them. For instance, while most yogurts are unacceptable during Induction, Hood Carb Countdown yogurt is one brand that is suitable. Moreover, private label products and those that are sold in only certain parts of the country are not listed. If you come across a brand that you are not familiar with, check out the company's website. Most food companies provide complete nutritional information for their products on their websites, which can offer more details than we can give in a book of this size and scope.

It is worth noting again that this book makes no effort to be comprehensive in terms of listing *all* foods, regardless of carb content. (That would be a multi-volume effort we will leave to a sociologist exploring the bizarre eating habits of the wealthiest and most-prone-to-excess society in the history of the world. It would be a little difficult to take that book to the store with you!) We do not list foods that are clearly out of bounds: French fries, for example, and batter-dipped shrimp, and the thousands of unacceptable cookies, crackers, snacks, and convenience foods are excluded.

WHAT ARE NET CARBS?

Not all carbohydrates behave the same way in your body. Some, such as table sugar, raise your blood sugar; others, such as fiber, sugar alcohols, glycerine and organic acids, pass through your body without significantly impacting your blood sugar. When you do Atkins, you count only the grams of carbohydrate that impact your blood sugar, which are called *Net Carbs*. To calculate the Net Carbs in most products, simply subtract the grams of fiber from the total number of grams of carbohydrate. (On the Nutrition Facts label shown opposite, the 8 grams of dietary fiber are subtracted from 13 grams of total carbohydrates to yield 5 grams of Net Carbs.) In the case of controlled-carb products sweetened with glycerine or sugar alcohols (when quantities are listed on the label), subtract those as well. Atkins products always provide the number of grams of Net Carbs in the Atkins seal on the front of the package (see opposite). Other low-carb manufacturers may calculate Net Carbs (which are sometimes referred to as "effective carbs" or "impact carbs") differently, so be sure to check the Nutrition Facts panel on the back of the package. When using a conventional carb-gram counter, simply subtract the grams of fiber from the total grams. *Dr. Atkins' New Carb Gram Counter* has done the math for you.

PHASES: Each food product is coded to indicate the phases of Atkins for which it is appropriate (see "A Four-Phase Program" on page 21). Several factors determine the appropriate phases, as follows:

- The food itself or certain ingredients in it.
- The number of grams of Net Carbs per serving based on the serving size listed on the Nutrition Facts panel.

Nutrition Facts

Serving Size 1/2 Cup (56g)
Servings Per Container 6

Amount Per Serving

Calories 210   Calories from Fat 35

	% Daily Value*
Total Fat 3g	**5%**
Saturated Fat 0.5g	**3%**
Cholesterol 0mg	**0%**
Sodium 280mg	**11%**
Total Carbohydrate 13g	**5%**
Dietary Fiber 8g	**33%**
Sugars 2g	
Protein 29g	**58%**

Vitamin A 0%	•	Vitamin C 0%
Calcium 8%	•	Iron 20%
Thiamine 4%	•	Riboflavin 0%
Niacin 4%	•	Folate 2%

*Percent Daily Values are based on a 2,000 calorie diet. Your daily values may be higher or lower depending on your calorie needs:

		Calories:	2,000	2,500
Total Fat	Less than		65g	80g
Sat Fat	Less than		20g	25g
Cholesterol	Less than		300mg	300mg
Sodium	Less than		2,400mg	2,400mg
Total Carbohydrate			300g	375g
Dietary Fiber			25g	30g
Protein			50g	60g

Calories per gram:
Fat 9 • Carbohydrate 4 • Protein 4

*For those controlling their carbs, count only 5 grams of the 13 grams of the Total Carbs in this product. Subtract dietary fiber (8g) which has a minimal impact on blood sugar.
Learn more: www.atkins.com/netcarbs

- Whether a product is a main dish or meal substitute, or a side dish, snack, dessert, or condiment.

Depending upon your individual tolerance for carbohydrates, a particular food may or may not be suitable for you. We have been conservative in our categorization of foods appropriate for phases. So while some people can introduce fruits other than berries in Phase 2: Ongoing Weight Loss, only berries are listed as suitable for phases 2–4. (It's worth pointing out that several fruits that most people consider vegetables—avocado, olives, and tomatoes, for instance—are perfectly acceptable during Induction.) On the other hand, there are foods listed for phases 3 and 4 that may not be suitable for you if you have a low tolerance for carbs (see "Understanding Your Carb Threshold" on page 14). Or a food coded for the phase you are in may be one you can eat only rarely or in very small portions. In the interest of space, we list phases by number, instead of by name, as follows:

Phase 1: Induction
Phase 2: Ongoing Weight Loss
Phase 3: Pre-Maintenance
Phase 4: Lifetime Maintenance

Assuming that a food does not have ingredients that make it unacceptable for a phase, Net Carb counts for phases are as follows:

Main dishes or meal substitutes:
- **Induction:** 0–7 grams per serving
- **Ongoing Weight Loss:** 0–12 grams per serving
- **Pre-Maintenance and Lifetime Maintenance:** 0–18+ grams per serving

Side dishes, appetizers, condiments, desserts or snacks:
- **Induction:** 0–3 grams per serving
- **Ongoing Weight Loss:** 0–9 grams per serving

- **Pre-Maintenance and Lifetime Maintenance:** 0–10+ grams per serving

There are certain exceptions to these categories: Although Net Carb count is key, a few foods with less than 3 grams of Net Carbs are not appropriate for the first two weeks of the Induction phase, when cravings for sweets may not yet be under control. So controlled-carb candies and other treats sweetened with sugar alcohols, for example, are not coded for Induction, no matter how low their Net Carb count. (Note that some people find that sugar alcohols can cause gastrointestinal distress and may want to limit their servings). Sugar alcohols include maltitol, isomalt, lactitol, and sorbitol. Glycerine is in the same family of ingredients.

Likewise, some people find that eating nuts and seeds in the first two weeks of Induction interferes with weight loss. Although nuts are low in carbohydrates, and some nut products contain less than 3 grams of Net Carbs, they are coded for phases 2–4. (Note that the small amount of nuts or dried berries in Atkins Advantage and Morning Start Bars is not enough to interfere with weight loss.) However, if you are allergic to peanuts or other nuts, be aware that all Advantage and Morning Start Bars and Endulge Chocolate Candies could have traces of nuts in them.

We used round numbers for grams of Net Carbs in keeping with Nutrition Facts panels, but the USDA numbers for vegetables and fruits, which include decimals, to be consistent with *Dr. Atkins' New Carb Gram Counter*.

SERVING SIZE: Our policy is to follow the United States Department of Agriculture (USDA) guidelines for servings of whole foods such as vegetables and fruits. With packaged foods, this is also typically the serving size listed on the Nutrition Facts panel. (Depending on category, some portion sizes are regulated by the Food and Drug Administration, or FDA.) Occasionally, when an indicated portion seems unreasonably small or large, such as shallots, which are used as a seasoning rather than as a vegetable, we have adjusted the portion size. Note that we are not specifying these serving sizes; it is up to you to keep track of your total Net Carb count and follow the guidelines of the ANA.

UNDERSTANDING YOUR CARB THRESHOLD

There are two numbers that you must learn to calculate to lose weight on Atkins permanently:

CCLL: When you do Atkins, instead of counting calories, you count the number of grams of carbs you consume each day. Once you are past phase 1, and while you are still in the process of losing weight, the carb gram count you are aiming for each day is known as your *Critical Carbohydrate Level for Losing* or CCLL. This is the number of grams of Net Carbs you can consume and still continue to lose weight. Your CCLL typically increases as you home in on your goal weight and deliberately slow down your weight-loss pace.

ACE: Once you have reached your goal weight and are maintaining it or are doing Atkins purely for health reasons, your "magic" number is known as your *Atkins Carbohydrate Equilibrium* or ACE. Your ACE represents the number of grams of Net Carbs you can consume each day while neither losing nor gaining weight.

➤ INGREDIENT ALERTS ◄

The beauty of doing Atkins is that there are so many delicious foods you can eat, allowing for the variety of tasty food necessary to make it a permanent lifestyle. This book is primarily about all the things you can eat. However, there are certain foods and ingredients you should try to avoid. Understand that an occasional portion of any individual food will likely not hurt you and an occasional lapse will likely not set you back; nonetheless, our goal is to provide you with this information to make it easier for you to adhere to the Atkins Nutritional Approach.

There are two categories of ingredients that are unacceptable at *any* phase of Atkins, even once you have slimmed down to your goal weight. Refined sugar is at the heart of the epidemics of obesity and diabetes that are undermining the health of a growing number of Americans; trans fats in the form of hydrogenated and partially hydrogenated oils have been shown to lead to heart disease. Neither of these foods has any place in the Atkins lifestyle.

ADDED SUGARS: Doing Atkins is not just about cutting down on carbs; equally important, it is about focusing on carbohydrate foods that are high in nutrients and fiber. For this reason, added sugars in any form are not acceptable at any phase of the program. Naturally occurring sugars, in dairy products (lactose) or in fruit (fructose), for instance, as well as in vegetables, are an organic part of the food, so they are acceptable if the carb count is within the appropriate range for a particular phase. An example: Low-carb ice cream has some naturally occurring sugars from the milk and cream from which it is made. If that ice cream has some strawberries (also natural sugars) in it, it could still be suitable for Ongoing Weight Loss and beyond. However, added fructose, sometimes used in food products in lieu of table sugar (sucrose), would make ice cream unacceptable in any phase. When a food appears at first glance to be all right in terms of the Net Carb count, but contains added sugars, it is marked with the "Ingredient Alert" symbol **A**, indicating it is an unacceptable food, with the words "Contains added sugars." Phases are omitted because the food should not be eaten at any phase of Atkins.

TRANS FATS: While fats from a variety of sources are integral to doing Atkins and to good health in general, there is one kind of fat that is dangerous. Manufactured trans fats, which are usually listed on labels as hydrogenated or partially hydrogenated oils, are made from inexpensive vegetable oils that have been heavily processed to make them thicker and more stable. (Humans actually produce trace amounts of naturally occurring trans fats in the intestine, as do other animals; when it comes to food products, we are talking about *added* trans fats—and these should be avoided at all costs.) Their use allows foods that would otherwise go bad quickly to have a long shelf life. The hydrogenation process that transforms fats changes their chemical structure, making your body unable to identify and process them. After many years, the USDA and FDA have finally ceded to consumer demands that trans fats be labeled as such on Nutrition Facts panels; presently, they are lumped in with saturated fats. Atkins has always cautioned against added trans fats and Atkins products contain no hydrogenated or partially hydrogenated oils. By 2006, all product packaging must identify trans fats, which is likely to reduce their use significantly. Any food product that contains added trans fats is marked with the "Ingredient Alert" symbol **A** and the words "Contains trans fats."

Unacceptable at any phase of Atkins, regardless of the Net Carb count, these product listings do not include phases. Consumption of saturated fats, on the other hand, is perfectly safe in the context of a controlled-carbohydrate lifestyle.

➤ PROCEED WITH CAUTION ◄

Certain other ingredients should be used prudently:

MONOSODIUM GLUTAMATE: A preservative and flavor enhancer, MSG can cause water retention and headaches in sensitive individuals. To help you avoid MSG we marked foods that contain it with the **FYI** symbol and the words "Contains MSG."

NITRATES: These preservatives are used in bacon, cured ham, pepperoni and certain other meats, smoked fish and other products to produce an appealing color and inhibit the growth of germs, which could lead to food poisoning. We marked them with the **FYI** symbol to alert you to their presence. Consider alternatives whenever possible. For example, instead of bologna or liverwurst, you could opt for sliced turkey or roast beef.

Certain other ingredients, such as white flour, cornstarch, and aspartame, are also indicated with the **FYI** symbol.

➤ ADVANCES IN FOOD SCIENCE ◄

In recent years, advances in food science have helped broaden and improve the controlled-carb food category. Not only has that made doing Atkins easier, it means that you don't have to give up certain categories of food "forever," something few people are willing to do. For example, the use of sucralose (see "Sugar Substitutes" on page 19) enables both commercial and home bakers to make sweets that are suitable—in moderation—for Atkins followers. Sugar alcohols such as maltitol make it possible to enjoy a chocolate candy bar without having a carb blowout. The development of such products is consistent with the Atkins commitment to variety and choice instead of monotony and deprivation.

Another technological breakthrough allows the use of small amounts of white flour in baked goods. As a result, we have moderated our former stance that all white flour was unacceptable at any phase of Atkins. Just a few years ago if you were doing Atkins your only options were to avoid bread in the weight-loss phases and have an occasional slice of whole-grain bread when you were at or close to your goal weight. (Whole-wheat flour and products made entirely with whole grains, such as bread and breakfast cereals, are acceptable—and are so coded—for the later phases of Atkins.) Bread made with white flour was a no-no in any phase.

Fortunately, the picture has changed. Food scientists have found out how to bake bread that tastes good and has the texture you expect, yet does not significantly impact your blood sugar, meaning that even in Induction you can have a slice of toast for breakfast. One of the ways they have done this is by using flour in a variety of forms. So, for example, Atkins Bakery breads contain a small amount of unbleached enriched white flour, but the Net Carb count is just 3 grams per slice. Compare this to the 14 or more grams of Net Carbs in a slice of bread made completely from white flour.

Do not take this slight liberalization about white flour in a controlled-carb product to improve taste and texture as carte blanche to eat conventional products full of white flour or to order breaded dishes in restaurants. It is only acceptable to eat a food that contains a small amount of white flour if the Net Carb count is quantified and falls within acceptable limits. Our overall recommendation continues to rely primarily on whole-grain flours, which contain the nutrient-rich germ and fiber-rich bran.

On a food ingredient list, white flour may appear as refined white flour, wheat flour, refined wheat flour, enriched flour, patent flour, or simply flour. Unless the label says, "100% whole-wheat flour," you can assume the ingredient is white flour. Further, it may be unbleached or bleached. Our preference is unbleached flour. To make you aware of the inclusion of white flour, we have identified foods that contain it with the **FYI** symbol even if the Net Carb count appears within acceptable limits.

When you think of cornstarch, you probably conjure up that stuff in a yellow and blue box that Mom used to thicken gravy. But another product that has transformed commercial baking is resistant starch. Also known as resistant cornstarch or resistant maltodextrin, it is resistant to digestion and never releases its glucose into the blood stream. As a result, this ingredient has a negligible impact on blood sugar levels and therefore is not included in the

Net Carb count. Because the words used on the label may not specify the type of cornstarch, we have also included the FYI symbol for these products. Wheat gluten, which is basically the protein part of the wheat minus the carbohydrate and fat, is also a key to making controlled-carb bread products. It too has a negligible impact on blood sugar.

➤ SUGAR SUBSTITUTES ◄

Although our sugar substitute of choice is sucralose (marketed as Splenda), saccharin (marketed as Sweet'N Low and Sugar Twin and other generic brands), and acesulfame-K (marketed as Sweet One, Swiss Sweet, and Sunett) are other options. The FDA does not recognize the use of the herb stevia as a sweetener, although it can be sold in natural foods stores as a dietary supplement. When a low-carb food contains aspartame, we have used the FYI symbol and the words "Contains aspartame" so that you can make your own purchasing decision.

We will be frank with you. The stated purpose of this book is to make it easier for you to obtain foods that are Atkins-friendly, so you will find it easier than ever to succeed at living this healthy, balanced lifestyle. But we have another hidden agenda and we might as well come clean with it now: We want you to control your carbs, but we also want you to eat the best quality foods you possibly can, and that means primarily whole foods. Doing Atkins is not just a numbers game. Of course, you should continue to count your carbs—at least until it becomes second nature and you are easily maintaining your weight—but *quality* is as important as quantity. We hope this book will help you to enhance the quality of your diet and your enjoyment of a variety of delicious and wholesome foods, as well. Let us leave you with some crucial reminders:

- Find your individual carb threshold.
- Then use products to support your individualized threshold.

After all, at Atkins our goal is to change the way the world eats to promote good health—including your health. We believe that this book will play an important part in doing just that!

—*Atkins Health & Medical Information Services*

A Brief Look at the Atkins Nutritional Approach

➤ A FOUR-PHASE PROGRAM ◄

Millions of people doing Atkins confirm that Atkins works, as does a host of recent research studies. But doing Atkins is not the same as just "eating low carb." That's why we are taking this opportunity to very briefly outline the advantages of the Atkins Nutritional Approach™ (ANA™). As individuals, we all have our differences—our likes and our dislikes. One of the benefits of Atkins is that it can be personalized to suit your particular needs, like your tastes and your activity level, among other factors. Many people confuse Induction, the first phase of Atkins, which lasts for a minimum of two weeks, as the entire ANA. However, Atkins is actually a four-phase program that begins with a relatively strict phase, and then moves through gradual liberalization to a permanent way of eating. Here is a brief rundown of each phase:

Phase 1: Induction kick-starts your body into weight loss, switching from a glucose metabolism (fueled by carbohydrates) to one that primarily burns fat, including your own body fat, for energy. When you stop relying on glucose for energy, you stabilize your blood sugar, which typically eliminates symptoms such as fatigue, mood swings, brain fog, and cravings for high-carbohydrate foods. Do Induction for a minimum of 14 days, after which you should see significant weight-loss results.

You will eat liberally of combinations of fat and protein in the form of poultry, fish, shellfish, eggs and red meat, as well as pure, natural fat in the form of butter, mayonnaise, olive oil, safflower, sunflower and other unadulterated vegetable oils. You will also eat 20 grams of Net Carbs each day, mostly in the form of salad greens and other vegetables. You can eat three to four loosely packed cups of salad, or two cups of salad plus one cup of other vegetables.

Eat absolutely no wheat bread, pasta, grains, starchy vegetables or dairy products other than cheese, cream, or butter. The only fruits permissible are avocados, olives, and tomatoes, which most people consider vegetables. Do not eat nuts or seeds in the first two weeks. (If you stay on Induction beyond two weeks, you can add both seeds and nuts.)

You can eat up to two servings of controlled-carb foods, such as an Atkins Advantage Bar or Shake or a Morning Start Bar, or use products such as selected Atkins Quick Quisine Bread & Muffin Mixes, so long as your total daily intake does not exceed 20 grams of Net Carbs. However, it is prudent to avoid sweets and certain desserts in the first two weeks of Induction, even if they contain less than 3 grams of Net Carbs per serving. If you have a lot of weight to lose, you can safely stay on Induction for six months or more.

Phase 2: Ongoing Weight Loss (OWL) lets you personalize the ANA to your tastes and needs, as you continue to burn fat and maintain control of your appetite sufficiently to control cravings. In this phase, you will gradually increase your consumption of carbs until you reach your threshold, known as your Critical Carbohydrate Level for Losing (CCLL), which will allow you to continue to lose weight. You will be able to eat a broader range of healthy foods, selecting those you enjoy most from a range of nutrient-rich carbohydrate foods as you deliberately slow your rate of weight loss to lay the groundwork for permanent weight management. To establish your CCLL, increase your daily carb intake by 5 grams of Net Carbs per week, so long as weight loss continues. When you stop losing weight for a week, drop back 5 grams and you should have found your carb threshold.

In OWL, most people can add more vegetables, fresh cheeses, nuts and seeds, berries, and low-carb specialty foods. Some people are able to add foods that are typically added in Pre-Maintenance. Foods should be introduced one at a time, to ensure that they do not create cravings, increase your appetite, cause weight gain or reintroduce old symptoms that disappeared in Induction. Continue doing OWL until you have 5 to 10 pounds left to lose.

Phase 3: Pre-Maintenance—In Ongoing Weight Loss, you increase your daily carb intake in increments of 5 grams per week. In this phase, increases in daily Net Carb count are in 10-gram increments each week as long as weight loss continues, albeit more slowly than in OWL. If new foods are introduced slowly and Net Carb grams increase gradually, your CCLL should slowly rise. During this phase most people can add legumes, fruit other than berries, higher-carb vegetables such as winter squash, carrots, peas and sweet potatoes, and finally whole grains. As you continue to make 10-gram incremental additions per week, you'll quickly reach a point at which you will find that you are no longer losing. If you are at your goal weight, stay at that level for a month or so before you increase your daily carb consumption by another 10 grams to see if you can consume at that level without gaining. Once you do begin to gain, drop back 10 grams and you should have established your Atkins Carbohydrate Equilibrium (ACE).

However, if after an incremental increase you find that you are gaining weight, or are not losing, and you are not yet at your goal weight, you'll need to back down to the previous level. The line between gaining, maintaining, and losing is a thin one, and you may have to play with your revised CCLL and ACE for a while to understand what your body can handle.

While it may take as long as three months to drop the last few pounds and clearly establish your ACE, this leisurely pace is critical to your ultimate success. Continue to add new foods slowly and carefully so you'll be learning good eating habits at the same time. (People with extremely low carb thresholds won't be able to add many new foods and will find Pre-Maintenance similar to Ongoing Weight Loss.)

Phase 4: Lifetime Maintenance—Once you have maintained your goal weight for a minimum of one month, you are officially in Lifetime Maintenance. You can continue to select from a greater range of foods and consume more carbs than you did in the weight-loss phases of the ANA. If your metabolism can handle it, you can—in moderation—eat many of the foods you used to enjoy. (The exceptions are sugar and bleached white flour.) Stay right at or around your ACE and your weight should not fluctuate beyond the perfectly natural range of 2 or 3 pounds. (Hormonal changes and other daily fluctuations in your body account for a small seesaw effect.)

For complete information on how to do Atkins, refer to *Dr. Atkins' New Diet Revolution.* If you have just a few pounds to lose, want to maintain your weight, or are interested in the health benefits of doing Atkins, refer to *Atkins for Life.* The newly published *The Atkins Essentials* focuses heavily on the first two weeks of doing Atkins. You can also find additional support at *www.atkins.com.*

➤ A NEW LOOK AT THE FOOD GUIDE PYRAMID ◄

Atkins Health & Medical Information Services recently developed an alternative food guide pyramid (see opposite) which emphasizes the importance of healthy protein sources, with vegetables as the primary source of carbohydrates. It also incorporates exercise as a key component of a healthy lifestyle.

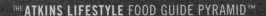

THE **ATKINS LIFESTYLE** FOOD GUIDE PYRAMID™

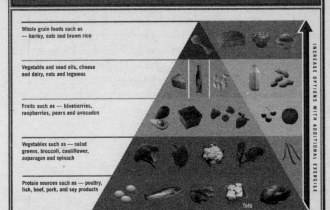

Whole grain foods such as
— barley, oats and brown rice

Vegetable and seed oils, cheese
and dairy, nuts and legumes

Fruits such as — blueberries,
raspberries, pears and avocados

Vegetables such as — salad
greens, broccoli, cauliflower,
asparagus and spinach

Protein sources such as — poultry,
fish, beef, pork, and soy products

Tofu

INCREASE OPTIONS WITH ADDITIONAL EXERCISE

HERE'S WHAT YOU DO: NO ADDED SUGARS & HYDROGENATED OILS

1. Limit and control certain carbohydrates to achieve and maintain a healthy weight.
2. Choose carbohydrates wisely (vegetables, fruits, legumes, whole grains), avoiding refined carbohydrates
   and foods with added sugars.
3. Eat until you are satisfied:
   - *to maintain weight, eat in proportion to the pyramid.*
   - *to lose weight, focus on protein, leafy vegetables and healthy oils.*
4. Everyone's metabolism and lifestyle are different. Discover your individual carb level to achieve and
   maintain a healthy weight. Raise this level with additional exercise.

PART 1:
THE SUPERMARKET
➤ **THE PERIMETER** ◄

The layout varies from store to store, but most often you'll find fresh foods—vegetables and fruits, meat, poultry, and dairy—on the outer walls of the store. When you're doing Atkins and following a controlled-carbohydrate lifestyle, this is where you should do the bulk of your shopping.

The Produce Aisle

Walk into any supermarket and the first thing you see is produce. It's no accident that bounteous displays of brightly colored vegetables and fruits greet you: Your first impression is surely one of variety, freshness, and healthful, wholesome foods. These are the core carbohydrate foods you will be eating on the Atkins Nutritional Approach™.

Vegetables and fruits, of course, are the bulk of the produce aisle, but some supermarkets also stock soy-based foods, like tofu, soy cheese and vegetarian hot dogs, here (often near organic produce), as well as Asian specialties like wonton wrappers. You might find imported cheeses, cured meats, and bakery breads and crackers, and perhaps an olive bar, in this area, too.

The problem with produce is that almost nothing bears a Nutrition Facts label. Unless you're armed with a carbohydrate gram counter, you have no sure way of knowing how many grams of Net Carbs are in a particular food. And while most vegetables are acceptable at all phases of Atkins, starchy ones such as sweet potatoes and peas, and most high-glycemic fruits (those that cause a greater rise in blood sugar), are usually added back only during the Pre-Maintenance and Lifetime Maintenance phases—unless you're one of the lucky folks with a high Critical Carbohydrate Level for Losing (CCLL) who can introduce them during OWL (see "Fruits and Vegetables: What's the Difference?" on page 54).

Because most produce lacks packaging with descriptive

copy about the vegetable or fruit, recipes, tips on how to cook it, or nutritional benefits, we'll go into more detail for foods in this section.

➤ VEGETABLES ◄

With few exceptions, the vast majority of vegetables can be enjoyed at any phase of Atkins. If you're not sure, go for the parts of plants that grow above ground. Roots and tubers like carrots and potatoes provide energy for growing plants, so they're usually higher in carbohydrates than leaves (lettuce, kale), flowers (broccoli florets, asparagus), and "fruit" or seed containers (tomato, zucchini, pepper). Vegetables that fall into the leaves, flowers, and fruit categories are the most nutrient-dense carbohydrates and, in the early phases of the Atkins Nutritional Approach, they're the major source of carbs.

Another clue to choosing nutrient-rich vegetables is to reach for the darker, more deeply colored ones. Pigments in plants contain compounds that can promote health in a variety of ways (see "Phytochemicals" on page 35). If your grocery list includes a vegetable with pale flesh—zucchini, say—be sure to leave the skin on to maximize nutrition as well as flavor.

Get to know the incredible array of vegetables out there and experiment with using them in your meals. For recipes and meal ideas, visit *www.atkins.com*.

DARK, LEAFY GREENS

An important source of folate (think *foliage*), dark, leafy greens are low in calories and Net Carbs, and high in flavor and nutrients.

Beet Greens (Phases 1-4)
3.7 g Net Carbs per ½ cup cooked

If you purchase beets with the greens attached, separate

them when you get home and store them individually, as they lose nutrients if left intact. Beet greens are high in beta carotene, vitamin C, and iron; they provide some calcium, too. *(Note: While beet greens are perfectly acceptable for Induction and beyond, the beet root is not acceptable until the later phases of the ANA; see "Beets" on page 36.)*

Bok Choy (Phases 1-4)
0.2 g Net Carbs per ½ cup cooked
One of the many varieties of Chinese cabbage, this mild-tasting green is often found in the Asian vegetables section (usually near the tofu and wonton wrappers). Choose a head with lots of dark green leaves; the stems should be pearly white. Baby bok choy looks like its full-grown counterpart except its stems are greener, not white. This versatile vegetable can be chopped for a salad, or stir-fry it until the leaves wilt and the stems are tender. For a more flavorful side dish, braise it with soy sauce, rice wine vinegar, gingerroot and a touch of low-carb sweetener.

Chard (Phases 1-4)
1.8 g Net Carbs per ½ cup cooked
Chard is a member of the beet family; it's grown for its leaves and stems rather than its roots. Chard is an excellent source of beta carotene, vitamins C and E, and iron. If you're taking an anticoagulant medication, opt for a different dark green leafy vegetable, since chard is also high in vitamin K, which can interfere with drugs that prevent blood clotting.

Collard Greens (Phases 1-4)
2 g Net Carbs per ½ cup cooked
Collard greens are high in folate and beta carotene, but they're particularly high in calcium—½ cup cooked weighs in at 113 milligrams of this essential mineral.

Dandelion Greens (Phases 1-4)
1.8 g Net Carbs per ½ cup cooked

Related to the sunflower, dandelion greens are indeed the same at the market as they are in your yard and a delightful addition to a salad of mixed greens. Unless you're certain your yard is untouched by pesticides and fertilizers, play it safe and go with the ones at the store. Choose small leaves; they become bitter as they grow.

Kale (Phases 1-4)
2.1 g Net Carbs per ½ cup cooked

Many types of kale exist, but the most common is curly kale. This dark green leafy vegetable is remarkably high in beta carotene, as well as the carotenoids lutein and zeaxanthin. Kale tastes somewhat sweeter after it's been exposed to frost, so purchase it in the winter. Choose bunches with slender stems—they're younger and milder in flavor.

Mustard Greens (Phases 1-4)
0.1 g Net Carbs per ½ cup cooked

This crucifer looks like smaller, brighter kale, but its flavor is much more assertive. Mustard greens are high in calcium, folate, and beta carotene.

Napa Cabbage (Phases 1-4)
0 g Net Carbs per ½ cup cooked

Another Chinese cabbage, this is likely to be near the bok choy and other Asian vegetables. Where bok choy is dark green and white, with a loose head, napa is pale green, somewhat rounded, and has crinkly leaves. You can eat it raw—simply slice it very thinly and toss with dark sesame or miso-style dressing for an Asian-style slaw. Or, cut into half-inch slices and stir-fry, then combine with soy sauce, rice vinegar and pepper flakes for a zesty side dish.

Turnip Greens (Phases 1-4)
0.6 g Net Carbs per ½ cup cooked

Turnip greens have a very pronounced flavor, but it's worth it to develop a taste for them: They provide exceptional amounts of beta carotene, vitamin C, folate, calcium, and iron.

CRUCIFEROUS VEGETABLES

These esteemed vegetables are part of the crucifer family because they contain substances that may protect against certain cancers. Cruciferous vegetables include the leafy greens collard, kale, and watercress, as well as the following:

Broccoflower (Phases 1-4)
2.3 g Net Carbs per ½ cup cooked
A hybrid of broccoli and cauliflower, this pale green vegetable shares cauliflower's milder taste but is higher in beta carotene.

Broccoli (Phases 1-4)
0.8 g Net Carbs per ½ cup raw; 1.7 g per ½ cup cooked
Broccoli supplies generous amounts of vitamin C, folate, beta carotene and iron. It's also high in sulfur compounds that fight cancer. Choose dark, rather than bright, green broccoli for higher amounts of beta carotene and vitamin C. Look at broccoli stems and avoid any that have a white core: It's lignin, a woody substance that's hard to chew.

Broccoli Rabe (Phases 1-4)
2 g Net Carbs per ½ cup raw
Botanically, this Italian vegetable is closer to turnips (rapa) than to broccoli; its seeds are used to make canola oil. Broccoli rabe doesn't keep as well as broccoli or other members of the brassica family, so don't store it for more than a few days.

Broccolini (Phases 1-4)
5 g Net Carbs per 8 stalks

A hybrid that's mostly broccoli with some Chinese broccoli and Chinese kale, broccolini (sometimes called baby broccoli) is crunchier and more delicately flavored than broccoli. Select the smallest spears you can find—they'll be indescribably tender.

Brussels Sprouts (Phases 1-4)
4.7 g Net Carbs per ½ cup cooked

High in vitamin C, folate, fiber, and carotenoids like lutein and zeaxanthin, Brussels sprouts are also surprisingly high in protein. Select those that are bright or deep green (avoid yellowish ones) and very small—they'll be the most tender. Look for them from mid-fall to early winter.

Cabbage (Phases 1-4)
- **Green** *1.1 g Net Carbs per ½ cup raw, shredded*
- **Red** *1.4 g Net Carbs per ½ cup raw, shredded*
- **Savoy** *1.9 g Net Carbs per ½ cup steamed*

The three main varieties include the largish green, the crinkly leaved Savoy, and the smaller red. All are rich in indoles and isothiocyanates, powerful antioxidants that are thought to prevent certain types of breast and prostate cancers. Of the three, red cabbage is highest in vitamin C, and it also contains anthocyanins, a group of antioxidant pigments.

Cauliflower (Phases 1-4)
0.9 g Net Carbs per ½ cup cooked

Unlike most vegetables, size doesn't matter with cauliflower. Select one based on how many servings you need, but be sure to choose one without brown spots. Cauliflower is high in vitamin C and should be steamed or roasted, rather than boiled, to get the most of this nutrient.

Kohlrabi (Phases 1-4)
4.6 g Net Carbs per ½ cup cooked

Kohlrabi peaks during the summer months. The round stems can be enjoyed raw (use like cucumbers, or thinly slice and smear with a soft cheese for an hors d'oeuvre) or boiled and mashed as you would potatoes. The leaves can be cooked like collards or kale.

Radishes (Phases 1-4)
1 g Net Carbs per ½ cup raw

Like other cruciferous vegetables, radishes are high in cancer-fighting compounds. In addition to the common red globe radishes, look for daikon radishes. They're long (18 inches isn't unusual), white, and can be somewhat football-shaped; daikon radishes have a sweet, fresh flavor.

PHYTOCHEMICALS

Wondering what exactly "phytochemicals" are? They're compounds in plants (*phyto* is from the Greek word for plant). Although thousands of these compounds have been identified, researchers are still discovering them—and what they are capable of doing.

Some phytochemicals are antioxidants, which means that they prevent unstable oxygen molecules from damaging cells. Others are thought to prevent cancer cells from forming, and others are thought to produce enzymes that neutralize carcinogens. Still others are thought to lower blood cholesterol or boost the immune system.

Many phytochemicals are found in the pigments of plants: Carotenoids, as you might suspect, give foods an orange or deep yellow hue. Exception: Some green vegetables are high in carotenoids, but the orange is masked by chlorophyll; anthocyanins give foods a blue or reddish color. Other phytochemicals are from elements like nitrogen or sulfur.

Sauerkraut (Phases 1-4)
2.1 g Net Carbs per ½ cup
If you've previously relied upon sauerkraut in cans or jars (see page 204), seek out bags in the refrigerator section of the produce department (they may also be near cured meats). It's less salty, and its crisp texture is more akin to freshly made sauerkraut.

ROOTS AND TUBERS

The rule of thumb for deeply colored vegetables is true of roots as well: Beets and carrots come out winners over potatoes and parsnips in the nutrition game.

Beets (Phases 3 & 4)
6.8 g Net Carbs per ½ cup cooked
Beets are higher in sugar than any other fresh vegetable, but their high fiber content helps to bring their Net Carb levels in line. Beet roots are an excellent source of folate—considerably higher than their greens—and provide some iron; their characteristic crimson color comes from betacyanin, an antioxidant pigment.

Burdock (Phases 3 & 4)
12.1 g Net Carbs per ½ cup cooked
Known as *gobo* in Japan, burdock has a slightly sweet, mild flavor if cooked—it can be quite bitter eaten raw.

Carrots (Phases 3 & 4)
5.6 g Net Carbs per ½ cup cooked
You can work carrots into your meals as soon as you're in Pre-Maintenance—but be sure to cook or serve them with butter or oil. Carrots are sky-high in beta carotene, a fat-soluble antioxidant, so fat helps your body absorb and use it.

Casava (Phases 3 & 4)
25.1 g Net Carbs per ½ cup cooked

This root (which also goes by the names manioc and yuca) is almost pure carbohydrate. It's common in Latin and African countries.

Celeriac (Phases 1-4)
3.6 g Net Carbs per ½ cup cooked

From a variety of celery grown for its root rather than its ribs, celeriac is round, rough, and covered with rootlets. Its texture is not unlike potatoes—use chunks in a beef stew or thin slices in a gratin. Choose comparatively smooth roots, which are easier to peel.

Gingerroot (Phases 1-4)
3.8 g Net Carbs per ¼ cup; 0 g per teaspoon

Gingerroot, like garlic, is used more as a flavoring than a vegetable, and like garlic it has a long history as a medicine. Look for smooth, glossy rhizomes, and unless you know you'll use a large piece within a month, choose a fairly small knob. Gingerroot will stay fresh for only a few weeks.

Jerusalem Artichoke (Phases 3 & 4)
11.9 g Net Carbs per ½ cup raw

Neither from Israel nor related to artichokes, this member of the sunflower (*girasole* in Italian) family is exceptionally high in iron.

Jicama (Phases 1-4)
2.5 g Net Carbs per ½ cup raw

Crisp, juicy, and somewhat sweet, thin slivers of this tuber add a wonderful crunch to salads, or add it to a beef-and-ginger stir-fry.

Parsnips (Phases 3 & 4)
12.1 g Net Carbs per ½ cup cooked

Despite their pale color, parsnips are fairly high in folate; they also supply vitamin C. Larger ones are fibrous, so look for those that are 6 to 8 inches long.

Potatoes (Phases 3 & 4)
10.5 g Net Carbs per ½ baked potato

Although potatoes contain vitamin C, you can't count on getting significant amounts from this vegetable since heat destroys this vitamin. And while potatoes are acceptable for later phases of Atkins, their high-glycemic index can result in unstable blood sugar, so eat them only rarely and in small portions.

Rutabaga (Phases 2-4)
5.9 g Net Carbs per ½ cup cooked

Fairly high in Net Carbs, rutabagas provide vitamin C and beta carotene. Buy the smallest ones you can find; they're sweeter and milder in flavor.

Sweet Potatoes (Phases 3 & 4)
12.1 g Net Carbs per ½ baked potato

An excellent source of beta carotene, vitamin E, vitamin C, and iron, sweet potatoes are a concentrated source of carbs. If you're craving something sweet, they're a good option (provided you're at least in Pre-Maintenance). But don't eat them mashed (36.9 g Net Carbs per ½ cup), which concentrates the amount of carbs, or candied (25 g Net Carbs per ½ cup).

Taro (Phases 3 & 4)
19.5 g Net Carbs per ½ cup

A tuber from the tropics, taro is very similar to potatoes in flavor and texture. It supplies some vitamin A.

Turnips (Phases 1-4)
2.3 g Net Carbs per ½ cup cooked, cubed; 3.3 g mashed

Like rutabagas (to which they're closely related), turnips supply vitamin C, but unlike rutabagas they provide no carotenoids. Choose smaller turnips (they're sweeter) and cut off the greens when you get home. Store the root and greens separately to retain vitamins.

SALAD GREENS

Whether you choose a mixture of loose greens, bags of salad blends, or a head of lettuce, salad greens are your major source of carbohydrate during Induction. Avoid bagged "salad kits"—they can include croutons or high-carb salad dressings and often dish out 6 grams of Net Carbs per serving.

Arugula (Phases 1-4)
0.2 g Net Carbs per ½ cup

Arugula isn't as high in nutrients as other salad greens—looseleaf and mâche are higher in beta carotene; looseleaf is higher in folate and vitamin C, too—but its peppery bite adds a sharp note to salads.

Endive (Phases 1-4)
0.4 g Net Carbs per ½ cup

Members of the endive family include escarole, curly endive (when small, it's called frisée), Belgian endive, radicchio. All but Belgian endive are good sources of vitamin C, vitamin E, folate, and beta carotene.

Escarole (Phases 1-4)
0 g Net Carbs per ½ cup

A member of the endive family, escarole is mild enough to add to salads, but is hardy enough to withstand cooking.

Lettuce (Phases 1-4)
- **Boston/Bibb** *0.4 g Net Carbs per ½ cup*
- **Iceberg** *0.2 g Net Carbs per ½ cup*
- **Looseleaf** *0.5 g Net Carbs per ½ cup*
- **Mesclun** *0.5 g Net Carbs per ½ cup*
- **Romaine** *0.2 g Net Carbs per ½ cup*

When building a salad, opt for darker greens—including those that are on the outside of the head of lettuce. Darker greens are higher in chlorophyll, which is linked to higher levels of beta carotene; they tend to have more vitamin C and folate, too.

Radicchio (Phases 1-4)
0.7 g Net Carbs per ½ cup

Radicchio is a member of the chicory family. It's often added to salad blends, but it can be cooked, too: Try braising or roasting it. Choose firm radicchio with absolutely no browning.

ALL ABOUT HERBS

Herbs contain generous amounts of nutrients, but they're rarely eaten in sufficient quantity to provide significant amounts. Likewise, when used as seasonings or garnish, they add virtually no grams of carbs to foods, so they can be used in all four phases of Atkins.

In addition to adding flavor to your recipes, fresh herbs can be added to salads—toss basil or parsley leaves into a green salad and taste what it does. Consider making herb sauces like pesto to maximize the vitamins these plants contain. Herbs also contain generous amounts of nutrients like folate, vitamin C, and beta carotene, and some supply iron. Experiment with the following herbs to enhance your favorite dishes without boosting carbs:

- Basil
- Chives
- Cilantro
- Dill
- Mint

- Oregano
- Parsley
- Rosemary
- Sage
- Thyme

Sorrel (Phases 1-4)
0.2 g Net Carbs per ½ cup

More common in European cuisines than American cooking, sorrel is often used in soups and sauces. Its tart flavor makes it a wonderful addition to a blend of salad greens.

Spinach (Phases 1-4)
0.1 g Net Carbs per ½ cup
Spinach is related to chard and beets. High in beta carotene and lutein and zeaxanthin, spinach is best served with an oil-based salad dressing or sautéed in oil—these carotenoids are fat-soluble, which means that the body is better able to absorb them in the presence of fat.

Watercress (Phases 1-4)
0 g Net Carbs per ½ cup
Like other cruciferous vegetables, watercress contains phytochemicals, particularly isothiocyanates and carotenoids.

LEGUMES

Although "legumes" are often referred to as dried beans, the term is more accurately used to describe the seed-bearing pods and the seeds of a type of plant. Information on dried beans can be found on page 235; canned beans on page 210; and heirloom beans available in natural foods stores on page 339.

Beans, Snap (green and wax) (Phases 1-4)
2.9 g Net Carbs per ½ cup cooked
Whether you choose green or the less common yellow wax beans, the taste and texture are the same; green beans are higher in folate and beta carotene.

Fava Beans (Phases 3 & 4)
12.1 g Net Carbs per ½ cup cooked
Also called broad beans, favas look like big lima beans. Look for fresh favas (usually in the pods) in late spring and early summer.

Peas, in pods (Phases 1-4)
3.4 g Net Carbs per ½ cup cooked

Snow peas and sugar snap peas are similar—snow peas are flatter and sometimes broader, with smaller peas inside; sugar snaps are rounder and have larger peas. Snow peas are very high in vitamin C, and supply folate, lutein and zeaxanthin.

Peas, shelled (Phases 3 & 4)
8.1 g Net Carbs per ½ cup cooked

If your only experience with green peas is limited to those from the freezer, look for fresh peas from mid-spring to early summer. Don't remove them from the shell until you plan to eat them—if they're very young and fresh, they don't even need to be cooked—but they don't store well, so use them the day you buy them.

Soybeans, fresh (Phases 3 & 4)
6.2 g Net Carbs per ½ cup cooked

Sometimes called edamame, fresh soybeans are an excellent source of thiamin, folate and iron. While they are not technically a complete protein, they do supply most of the essential amino acids needed by the human body.

MUSHROOMS

Mushrooms are an excellent way to add a range of flavors to many foods: They contain glutamic acid, a natural compound on which the flavor enhancer monosodium glutamate (MSG) is based. Look beyond plain white mushrooms—cremini (sometimes called baby bellas), portobellos, and shiitake mushrooms add a little something extra to dishes.

Mushrooms (Phases 1-4)
- **Button (white)** *1.4 g Net Carbs per ½ cup raw, whole*
- **Cremini** *3.9 g Net Carbs per ½ cup raw, whole*
- **Portobello** *4.1 g Net Carbs per 4-ounce mushroom*
- **Shiitake** *8.8 g Net Carbs per ½ cup cooked*

SUMMER SQUASH

Do consider size when you're shopping for squash. Choose the smallest one you can find—it will have smaller seeds and a more delicate texture.

Chayote (Phases 1-4)
1.8 g Net Carbs per ½ cup cooked
Related to cucumber and zucchini, chayote tastes like a combination of both. It goes by many names, including mirliton in Caribbean and Creole cooking, and is used in Chinese cuisine. Use it, cooked or not, as you would zucchini (though it needs to be cooked longer).

Pattypan (Phases 1-4)
1.3 g Net Carbs per ½ cup cooked
Sometimes called scallop squash, pattypan is about the size of a hockey puck, with scalloped edges. Pale green in color, pattypan turns white as it matures.

Yellow Squash (Phases 1-4)
1.4 g Net Carbs per ½ cup raw; 2.6 g ½ cup cooked
Look for crookneck and straightneck, which looks like yellow zucchini. Yellow squash supplies about one-tenth the lutein and zeaxanthin than zucchini does.

Zucchini (Phases 1-4)
1.1 g Net Carbs per ½ cup raw; 1.5 g ½ cup cooked
This most common summer squash is a good source of vitamin C (cooking destroys it, so raw squash provides more) and fiber. Leave the skin on to obtain the carotenoids—zucchini's peel is very high in lutein and zeaxanthin.

WINTER SQUASH

Most winter squash are a superb source of fiber, potassium, beta carotene, and vitamin C, and supply respectable amounts of folate, vitamin E, and B vitamins. They also supply alpha carotene and lutein.

Acorn Squash (Phases 3 & 4)
10.4 g Net Carbs per ½ cup baked; 7.6 g ½ cup boiled

High in fiber and beta carotene, acorn squash also supplies generous amounts of thiamin, vitamin C, iron, potassium, folate, and vitamin E.

Butternut Squash (Phases 3 & 4)
7.9 g Net Carbs per ½ cup baked;
9.4 g ½ cup baked, then mashed

Butternut squash is an excellent source of beta carotene and vitamin C.

Hubbard Squash (Phases 1-4)
4.2 g Net Carbs per ½ cup boiled

These blue-gray squash tend to be enormous, so you may find them precut in your market.

Pumpkin Squash (Phases 1-4)
4.6 g Net Carbs per ½ cup cooked

If you need mashed pumpkin, it's much easier to use canned—it's been cooked down enough so that it won't become watery in most recipes. (Just be sure to use 100% pumpkin puree, not pumpkin pie filling, which contains sugar.) Otherwise, use pumpkin as you would any other winter squash. It's very high in carotenoids, particularly beta carotene, alpha carotene, and lutein.

Spaghetti Squash (Phases 1-4)
3.9 g Net Carbs per ½ cup cooked

Preparing spaghetti squash tends to be time-consuming, but its similarity to strands of spaghetti is astonishing. Make some on the weekend and heat it up with your favorite pasta sauce.

OTHER VEGETABLES

Here are common vegetables that don't really fall into the previously mentioned categories:

Artichokes (Phases 1-4)
6.9 g Net Carbs per 1 medium; 4.9 g per ½ cup hearts

At their peak from March through May and in October, the best artichokes are compact and squeak when pressed or squeezed. Artichokes are very high in fiber, and provide iron, magnesium, and folate, too.

Asparagus (Phases 1-4)
1.6 g Net Carbs per 4 spears cooked;
1.9 g per ½ cup cooked

High in fiber, folate and flavor, asparagus comes into season in early spring. To choose the best, look at the bottoms of the stalks—avoid oval spears, which can be woody or tough, and go for those that are rounder. Thicker spears are actually more tender and juicy than thin ones.

Bamboo Shoots (Phases 1-4)
1.2 g Net Carbs per ½ cup cooked

It's unlikely that you'll find these fresh, unless you venture to supermarkets with a large Asian clientele. Bamboo must be cooked to be edible, but once it's cooked it can be used in place of jicama or water chestnuts in stir-fried dishes or salads.

Cardoon (Phases 1-4)
2.7 g Net Carbs per ½ cup cooked

Although cardoons are shaped like big celery, they aren't as bright or as crisp. Because large ones can be stringy, choose the smallest bunch with the slenderest ribs you can find. Look for them in markets in fall and winter.

Celery (Phases 1-4)
1.8 g Net Carbs per ½ cup cooked; 0.8 g per rib, raw

For the freshest, least-stringy celery, look for sprightly leaves and pale-green ribs. Celery is low in calories and carbs—one rib has a mere 6 calories—but don't believe the myth that it has "negative calories." Eating celery burns about 2 calories per minute.

Corn (Phases 3 & 4)
12.6 g Net Carbs per ½ cup cooked; 17.2 g per ear

More than 200 varieties of sweet corn are grown; choose corn with yellow, not white, kernels and you'll get lutein and zeaxanthin, two carotenoids that can protect against age-related eye disorders.

Cucumbers (Phases 1-4)
1.0 g Net Carbs per ½ cup raw, sliced

Relatives of summer squash, cucumbers are mostly water, so take care you don't store them in a super-cold refrigerator, lest they freeze. Don't peel them, as their skins are high in lutein, and choose small ones except for hothouse (or English) cukes—these can grow to be 18 inches long.

Eggplant (Phases 1-4)
2.1 g Net Carbs per ½ cup broiled

A good source of fiber and potassium, eggplant doesn't provide significant amounts of most vitamins. Whether you purchase baby eggplant, Japanese (long, thin, usually dark purple), Chinese (long, thin, usually white), American (the familiar rounded purple ones), or Italian (smaller version of American), choose small yet heavy eggplants.

Fennel (Phases 1-4)
1.5 g Net Carbs per ½ cup cooked; 1.8 g ½ cup raw

Fennel's subtle anise flavor and crisp texture are ideal raw (slice and use as dippers for a crudité platter) or cooked (sauté, braise, or roast it). The entire plant—seeds, fronds, stalks, and bulb—can be eaten. Fennel is best from early fall to spring.

Nopales (Phases 1-4)
1.0 g Net Carbs per ½ cup cooked

Sometimes called cactus pads, nopales have a mild flavor and crisp texture. Peel them, then steam and toss with lemon juice. Nopales are a good source of vitamin C.

Okra (Phases 1-4)
3.8 g Net Carbs per ½ cup cooked

High in vitamin C, lutein and zeaxanthin, and soluble fiber, okra can be hard to find outside of the South. Look for it in the summer, but if the pods are longer than 3 or so inches, they'll probably be less tender, so pass on them (look for frozen okra instead; see page 291).

Peppers, Chili (Phases 1-4)
- **Jalapeño** *1.4 g Net Carbs per ½ cup sliced*
- **Serrano** *1.6 g Net Carbs per ½ cup*
- **Ancho** *5.1 g Net Carbs per chili*
- **Pasilla** *1.7 g Net Carbs per chili*

You'll find fresh chilis like jalapeño, Serrano, poblano, even fiery habanero, as well as dried ones like ancho, chipotle, pasilla, chiles de arbol, in most stores. Chili peppers get their heat from capsaicin, a phytochemical so caustic that one drop, diluted in 100,000 drops of water, can blister the tongue. Peppers vary considerably in the amount of capsaicin they contain. As a very general rule, the smaller the pepper, the hotter it is.

Peppers, Sweet (Phases 1-4)
- **Green Bell** *3.5 g Net Carbs per ½ cup raw*
- **Red Bell** *3.3 g Net Carbs per ½ cup raw*
- **Yellow Bell** *2.8 g Net Carbs per 10 strips (slightly less than ½ cup)*

When it comes to peppers, "sweet" is something of a misnomer—these aren't sugary, they're just not hot. Although bell peppers are the most common sweet pepper, you may find Cubanelles (sometimes called Italian frying peppers), banana peppers, or pimientos. If you can, choose red rather than green peppers; they supply more than twice the vitamin C, and they contain beta carotene and beta cryptoxanthin.

Sprouts (Phases 1-4)
- **Alfalfa** *0.2 g Net Carbs per ½ cup*
- **Mung Bean** *2.1 g Net Carbs per ½ cup*
- **Broccoli** *0.8 g Net Carbs per ½ cup*

You may know bean sprouts from Chinese cooking, alfalfa sprouts as a salad topping, but have you tried broccoli sprouts? They are a highly concentrated source of sulforaphane, a sulfur compound full of cancer-fighting properties.

One word of caution about sprouts: According to the FDA, sprouts have been linked to 13 foodborne illness outbreaks since 1995, and many of these outbreaks have involved raw alfalfa sprouts. Children, the elderly and individuals with compromised immune systems should avoid raw alfalfa sprouts. Otherwise, take precautions when buying and using sprouts. Be sure to purchase only sprouts that have been kept refrigerated, are crisp looking and have their buds attached. Refrigerate sprouts when storing at home and rinse them thoroughly with water to remove surface dirt before using. And always wash hands well using warm water and soap before and after handling raw foods.

Tomatoes (Phases 1-4)
- **Cherry** *2.0 g Net Carbs per ½ cup*
- **Red** *2.5 g Net Carbs per ½ cup*
- **Plum** *1.7 g Net Carbs per tomato*

High in vitamin C, tomatoes have recently received

press for the generous amounts of the carotenoid lycopene they provide. (Canned or cooked tomatoes contain lycopene in higher concentrations.) Cherry and plum tomatoes provide some vitamin E. While they are technically considered fruits, tomatoes are commonly thought of as vegetables.

Tomatillos (Phases 1-4)
2.6 g Net Carbs per ½ cup
Tomatillos look like green cherry tomatoes in a papery husk. They are commonly used in salsa verde.

ALLIUMS

Garlic, leeks, onions and scallions are high in antioxidant sulfur compounds, which also give them their distinctive flavors.

Garlic (Phases 1-4)
0.9 g Net Carbs per clove
Used as a medicine since ancient times, modern science is proving that garlic has remarkable antioxidant powers. It contains allicin, a compound that develops when the vegetable is exposed to oxygen but not in the presence of heat. Try to chop or crush garlic 10 minutes before you cook it so the allicin has time to develop; once it has developed, heat won't destroy it.

Leeks (Phases 1-4)
3.4 g Net Carbs per ½ cup cooked
Though they're available year round, leeks are at their best (and least expensive) from autumn through spring. Choose smaller leeks—they're more tender—and clean them thoroughly before cooking. Try them baked: Arrange 1- to 2-inch lengths on a foil square; drizzle with olive oil, herbs, salt, and pepper. Seal the packet well and bake at 350 or 400 degrees until tender, 15–20 minutes.

Onions (Phases 1-4)
5.5 g Net Carbs per ½ cup raw; 5 g per ½ cup cooked
Sweet onions, such as Vidalia and Oso Sweet, are slightly lower in sugar than regular storage onions are (they're milder in flavor because they're lower in the compounds that make onions so pungent). Look for them in the spring and summer. During Induction, onions should be used primarily as a garnish.

Scallions (Phases 1-4)
2.4 g Net Carbs per ½ cup cooked
Scallions, also known as green onions, are immature onions. Their flavor is somewhat milder, and they are much more perishable, but they come with a nutritional bonus: Their green tops contain beta carotene. (Because raw scallions have been linked to outbreaks of Hepatitis A, the FDA suggests that concerned consumers cook scallions thoroughly and avoid foods containing raw scallions.)

Shallots (Phases 1-4)
3.1 g Net Carbs per 2 tablespoons cooked
Shallots look and taste like a cross between onions and garlic—and can be used as you would onions. With shallots, a little goes a long way.

➤ SOY-BASED AND ASIAN FOODS ◄

Most supermarkets stock several varieties of tofu, as well as soy foods like cheese, hot dogs and non-frozen veggie burgers in the refrigerator case of the produce section. You may find them near Asian vegetables and foods like wonton skins.

Soy protein contains isoflavones, plant compounds that have been linked to cardiovascular health, particularly lower levels of blood cholesterol, and are thought to alleviate symptoms of menopause and reduce the risk of cancers caused by hormonal irregularities.

If you don't have much experience cooking with, or eating, tofu, get started by purchasing soy-based cheese, or a meat analog (substitute) like "bacon," "sausage," "burgers" or "hot dogs," which are easier to incorporate into recipes and meals. Seek out low-carb recipes for tofu; we offer a slew of easy-to-prepare dishes at *www.atkins.com*. (For more information on soy foods, go to page 340.)

TOFU

Tofu, or soybean curd, is available in a variety of textures, from extra-firm to soft. Firm tofu is better for stir-fries and grilling because it retains its shape and texture. Soft tofu, on the other hand, works best for blending and adding to soups. You'll most often find tofu in water-packed tubs or aseptic boxes.

Flavored tofus are a good alternative for quick meals—you won't need to scrounge for spices or flavorings—but avoid those that come with sauces. Flavored tofu without sauce has about 2 grams Net Carbs per serving; those with a sauce can have 5–7 grams Net Carbs and contain added sugars.

Tofu, firm (Phases 1-4)
2 g Net Carbs per ⅕ block

Tofu, soft (Phases 1-4)
2 g Net Carbs per ⅕ block

Tempeh (Phases 1-4)
3.3 g Net Carbs per ½ cup
Made of cooked, fermented soybeans, tempeh is higher in protein than tofu is; it also has more flavor. Tempeh is always firm in texture.

Seitan (Phases 1-4)
2 g Net Carbs per piece
A meat substitute made from wheat gluten, seitan is high

in protein. Seitan has a chewy, firm texture that holds up well to stir-frying.

Tofu Hot Dogs, Bacon, and Sausage Links (Phases 1-4)
- **Tofu Hot Dogs** *2-5 g Net Carbs per dog*
- **Tofu Bacon** *2 g Net Carbs per 2 strips*
- **Tofu Canadian Bacon** *0 g Net Carbs per 3 slices*
- **Tofu Link Sausage** *4 g Net Carbs per 2 links*
- **Tofu Bulk Sausage** *2 g Net Carbs per 2 ounces*

In addition to supplying varying amounts of soy protein, these foods made from tofu have one distinct advantage over their meat-based counterparts: They are free from nitrates (see page 66). They also vary considerably in flavor between brands, so if you're not fond of one, try another.

Veggie Burgers, Crumbles, and Meatballs (Phases 1-4)
- **Burgers** *2 g Net Carbs per burger*
- **Crumbles** *2 g Net Carbs per ⅓ cup*
- **Meatballs** *4 g Net Carbs per 4–5 meatballs*

These are ideal substitutes for meatless meals. Always check package labels; Net Carbs and ingredients vary by brand.

Veggie Cheese (Phases 1-4)
- **Slices** *1 g Net Carb per slice*
- **Shredded** *2 g Net Carbs per serving*
- **Parmesan** *0.5 g Net Carbs per serving*
- **Cream Cheese** *2 g Net Carbs per serving*

Based on soybeans rather than milk, veggie cheese products can be lower in Net Carbs than dairy products.

> **WORST BITES:** Proof that vegetarian and natural aren't always nutritious, some meat substitutes can be higher in Net Carbs than their meat-based counterparts. Often, veggie wings are coated with a sweetened sauce, the nuggets are coated with breading, and the chili is high in beans.
>
> **Veggie Wings, Nuggets, and Chili**
> * **Wings** *17 g Net Carbs per 4 wings*
> * **Nuggets** *12–20 g Net Carbs per 4 nuggets*
> * **Chili** *23 g Net Carbs per 10½-ounce container*

➤ FRUITS ◄

Most fruits are acceptable in the Pre-Maintenance and Lifetime Maintenance phases of the Atkins Nutritional Approach. Because they are relatively low in carbohydrates (and have a high-antioxidant content), berries are among the first foods added back during Ongoing Weight Loss.

Also, when it's time to add other fruits back to your menus, do so slowly and in small increments. Revise your impression of fruit: Rather than considering it a snack, think of it as an ingredient. Count out a portion of grapes, then halve or quarter them and add them to a chicken salad. Cut half a peach into controlled-carb yogurt for a morning treat (give the other half to a family member, or wrap it up for another meal).

Although not traditionally considered fruits, olives and avocados, both of which are acceptable foods on Induction, are botanically considered fruits.

FRUITS AND VEGETABLES:
WHAT'S THE DIFFERENCE?

We associate fruits with sweetness and desserts; vegetables are more savory. But how else do they differ?

Vegetables are, most broadly, plants that are grown for edible parts, whether leaves, stems, roots, or even fruits. Fruits are the edible pulpy part of plants that surround seeds. So while everyone considers oranges and apples to be fruits, a botanist would tell you that tomatoes, avocados, peppers, and zucchini are fruits, too.

BERRIES

Berries are the first food you'll add back to your menus after Induction, and for good reason: They contain fabulously high concentrations of beneficial plant compounds and are fairly low in Net Carbs.

Blackberries (Phases 2-4)
5.4 g Net Carbs per ½ cup

High in soluble fiber, vitamin C, and phytochemicals, like anthocyanins and ellagic acid, blackberries are at their peak from late spring through mid-summer. Boysenberries, a variety of blackberries, have the same grams of Net Carbs per serving.

Blueberries (Phases 2-4)
8.3 g Net Carbs per ½ cup

Among the most antioxidant-rich foods, blueberries contain generous amounts of soluble fiber, vitamins E and C, as well as several types of anthocyanins. Cultivated blueberries are at their best in early summer (though they're available year-round), but keep an eye out for tiny and tasty wild blueberries.

Cranberries (Phases 2-4)
4 g Net Carbs per ½ cup raw

The good news about cranberries is that they're almost as nutrient-rich as blueberries. The bad news is they are so tart that they verge on unpalatable when raw and unsweetened. Try making cranberry sauce using sucralose to mellow their naturally tart flavor.

Currants (Phases 2-4)
5 g Net Carbs per ½ cup

These tiny berries are relatives of the gooseberry and can be found from June through August. Stir them into sauces or enjoy them sweetened with sucralose and topped with cream.

Gooseberries (Phases 2-4)
4.4 g Net Carbs per ½ cup

Like other berries, gooseberries are high in fiber and vitamin C, as well as in phytochemicals. Look for them from late May through July; use them in a pan sauce for sautéed chicken or salmon.

Loganberries (Phases 2-4)
5.4 g Net Carbs per ½ cup

A hybrid of blackberries and raspberries, loganberries are purplish-red and somewhat tart when ripe. Look for them in June and July. Loganberries are quite perishable, so use them within a day or two of purchase.

Raspberries (Phases 2-4)
3 g Net Carbs per ½ cup

Exceptionally high in flavor and fiber, these sweet morsels are at their best from late spring to mid-autumn. Handle them gently—they are incredibly fragile, and are best eaten as soon as possible after purchase. Red and black raspberries contain anthocyanins; the rarer gold ones don't.

Strawberries (Phases 2-4)
3.4 g Net Carbs per ½ cup, whole
Ounce for ounce, strawberries are higher in vitamin C than oranges. They contain anthocyanins and ellagic acid (an antioxidant), as well as fiber. Locally grown berries in season will be higher in flavor and freshness than shipped berries. Like all berries, strawberries are highly perishable.

CITRUS FRUITS

Pass on the juice (except for lemon and lime juice) and get your citrus from the fruit itself—you'll get significantly more fiber and, if you eat the membranes, phytochemicals.

Grapefruits (Phases 3 & 4)
- **Red** *7.9 g Net Carbs per ½ grapefruit*
- **White** *8.6 g Net Carbs per ½ grapefruit*

Best known for their vitamin C content, grapefruit—at least the red and darker pink ones—are high in beta carotene and lycopene, two carotenoids. Need more reasons to choose red? They're slightly higher in fiber and in vitamin C than the white, and they tend to be sweeter.

Kumquats (Phases 3 & 4)
7.5 g Net Carbs per 4 kumquats
These adorably small citrus fruits can be eaten, skin and all. They're most often in supermarkets from late autumn through March. Kumquats are high in vitamin C.

Lemons (Phases 1-4)
2.5 g Net Carbs per 2 tablespoons
Fresh lemon juice is vastly superior to bottled; it's worth it to keep a few fresh lemons on hand at all times. Choose lemons that feel heavy for their size—they contain more juice—and don't forget to use the zest, or yellow part of the peel, in recipes. It's high in limonenes, a phytochemical with anticancer properties.

Limes (Phases 1-4)
2.9 g Net Carbs per 2 tablespoons

The greener the lime, the tarter the juice—yellower limes are riper, and their juice can be bland. As with lemons, lime zest is high in limonenes.

Oranges (Phases 3 & 4)
8.4 g Net Carbs per ½ cup sections;
12.9 g per medium orange

High in vitamin C, oranges supply fiber and some folate, too. The most common oranges are navel and Valencia, but keep an eye out for blood oranges in the winter. They are very sweet and juicy, and their deep crimson color comes from anthocyanins, the pigments that give berries their antioxidant punch.

Tangerines (Phases 3 & 4)
6.2 g Net Carbs per small tangerine

Tangerines, with their close cousins clementines and mandarin oranges, contain vitamin C as well as a host of carotenoids: beta carotene, beta cryptoxanthin, lutein and zeaxanthin.

MELONS

Melons are high in antioxidants. Steer clear of precut melon at supermarkets—these fruits are high in vitamin C, which diminishes rapidly when exposed to oxygen. Buy whole fruits and slice them yourself to preserve the nutrients.

Cantaloupes (Phases 3 & 4)
6.7 g Net Carbs per ½ cup melon balls

An excellent source of vitamin C, beta carotene, and potassium.

Crenshaw Melons (Phases 3 & 4)
4.6 g Net Carbs per ½ cup melon balls

Crenshaw melons supply some beta carotene and vitamin C.

Honeydew Melons (Phases 3 & 4)
7.3 g Net Carbs per ½ cup melon balls
Honeydews supply generous amounts of vitamin C and zeaxanthin.

Watermelons (Phases 3 & 4)
5.1 g Net Carbs per ½ cup melon balls
Lycopene is associated with tomatoes, but watermelon is higher in this carotenoid than uncooked tomatoes are.

TROPICAL FRUITS

Thanks to improved methods of shipping, many of these fruits are available year-round, even in northern climes.

Avocados, Haas (Phases 1-4)
1.7 g Net Carbs per ½ avocado
Haas avocados are the smaller ones, with the dark, pebbly skin. They're considerably lower in Net Carbs than the larger, brighter Florida avocados (which have 5.5 g per ½ avocado), and they're higher in beneficial fats, making them a satisfying addition to Induction. Avocados are high in fiber, folate and iron.

Bananas (Phases 3 & 4)
21.2 g Net Carbs per small banana
Although an excellent source of vitamin B_6, bananas are also very high in Net Carbs. As bananas ripen, the starch turns to sugar. Once bananas are just barely ripe, store them in the refrigerator to prevent them from ripening further.

Coconut (Phases 1-4)
2.5 g Net Carbs per ½ cup
Obtaining fresh coconut meat can be a production, but it's worth the effort. These fruits supply some folate, and they're a good source of fiber and cholesterol-lowering phytosterols. (See page 217 for coconut milk.)

Kiwi (Phases 3 & 4)
8.7 g Net Carbs per kiwi

Exceptionally high in fiber, vitamin C, and potassium, kiwis also contain lutein and cholorogenic acid, two antioxidant phytochemicals. There's no need to peel a kiwi—not only are the skins edible, they're full of nutrients. Just wash and rub off the fuzz.

Mango (Phases 3 & 4)
12.5 g Net Carbs per ½ cup

Mangos range in color from green to gold to reddish orange; the color varies by type, not ripeness. A mango that's past its prime smells somewhat fermented and remains indented when pressed gently—choose fruits that smell flowery and spring back when pressed.

Papaya (Phases 3 & 4)
6.1 g Net Carbs per ½ small papaya

High in vitamin C, vitamin E, folate, and fiber, papaya also contains beta carotene and beta cryptoxanthin. Don't discard the seeds—they are edible and have a spicy, somewhat peppery flavor.

Passion Fruit (Phases 3 & 4)
7.7 g Net Carbs per ¼ cup

Because passion fruit is grown all over the world, it's available almost year-round. The most common type found in American markets is egg-shaped and has a purple rind. The seeds are edible and contribute a great deal of fiber to the fruit.

Pineapple (Phases 3 & 4)
8.7 g Net Carbs per ½ cup

Pineapples are harvested when they are on the verge of being fully ripe; the best-quality ones are shipped by air from tropical areas like Hawaii, Florida, and Central America. Choose large pineapples, as they have more succulent flesh compared to fibrous core. See page 172 for dried pineapple.

Plantains (Phases 3 & 4)
21 g Net Carbs per ½ cup

Popular in Latin American countries, plantains are a larger, firmer variety of banana, typically served cooked. The flavor is mild and similar to squash.

STONE FRUITS

Your best bet with stone fruits is to buy those that are locally grown at the height of their season. (See pages 170–173 for dried apricots, cherries, peaches and plums.)

Apricots (Phases 3 & 4)
9.2 g Net Carbs for 3 medium apricots

Apricots don't ship well, so if you live far from where they're grown you may have trouble finding them—or finding fragrant, exquisitely flavored ones. Don't settle for canned apricots: They are lower in beta carotene and vitamin C, and higher in sugars.

Cherries (Phases 3 & 4)
8.3 g Net Carbs per ½ cup sweet cherries

Although Bing cherries are the most commonly available commercial cherries, you may find other sweet cherries like Rainier, or sour cherries like Montmorency, in some markets. Cherries are in season from late spring to mid-summer. Choose Bing cherries carefully, looking for dark red fruit with unbroken skins.

Nectarines (Phases 3 & 4)
13.8 g Net Carbs per medium nectarine

In season throughout the summer months, nectarines are available with the familiar peachy-gold flesh and with a white flesh. Choose the yellow variety for the carotenoids it contains: beta carotene and beta cryptoxanthin.

Peaches (Phases 3 & 4)
7.2 g Net Carbs per small peach

At their peak in summer, peaches are best locally grown: Once they are picked, they don't get any sweeter. The best way to determine ripeness is by feeling and smelling—many peaches are bred to have a red blush to the skins no matter how ripe they are (or aren't). In addition to the common yellowy-pink peach, look for white peaches.

Plums (Phases 3 & 4)
3.3 g Net Carbs per small plum

Plums supply some vitamin C, as well as small amounts of vitamin E. Black, purple, and red plums are high in the antioxidants anthocyanins.

GRAPES

Grapes, particularly those with dark skins, supply a host of phytochemicals. Eat them with caution, though, because they're high in Net Carbs. (See page 173 for raisins.)

Grapes (Phases 3 & 4)
- **Green** *13.7 g Net Carbs per ½ cup*
- **Red** *13.4 g Net Carbs per ½ cup*
- **Purple Concord** *7.4 g Net Carbs per ½ cup*

If your preferred grape is green seedless, think about this: Seeded grapes are considered more flavorful than seedless varieties, and red and black grapes are thought to have higher levels of flavonoids like resveratrol and anthocyanins. Keep an eye out for American grapes like Concord and Scuppernong, as well as the small and exquisitely flavored Champagne grapes, in early fall.

OTHER FRUITS

Here are common fruits that don't fall into one of the previously mentioned categories:

Acerola (Phases 3 & 4)
3.2 g Net Carbs per ½ cup

Acerolas, small, dark red fruits similar to cherries, don't appear in markets too frequently, but they're worth keeping an eye out for because they're very high in vitamin C. They're most often used in desserts and preserves.

Apples (Phases 3 & 4)
8.7 g Net Carbs per ½ medium apple

Want to get the most nutrients out of your apple? Choose one with a red peel and eat the skins. Red apple peels contain anthocyanins; all apples contain quercetin. (See page 170 for dried apples).

Carambola (Star Fruit) (Phases 3 & 4)
2.8 g Net Carbs per ½ cup sliced

Originally from Asia, this fruit is now grown in Florida. Wait to eat carambola until the skin is a deep yellow gold color and aromatic. Star fruit provides some vitamin C.

Cherimoya (Phases 3 & 4)
24.3 g Net Carbs per ½ cup

Often called custard apple, cherimoyas are wonderfully fragrant and sweet. They're often stocked near jicama, plantains, and other Central American and Caribbean produce.

Dates (Phases 3 & 4)
16.4 g Net Carbs per 3 fresh dates

Available both fresh and dried, dates are high in carbohydrate—of those 16.4 g Net Carbs, 15.8 g are sugars. You're most likely to find deglet noor and medjools in supermarkets. Snip them (it's easier than chopping) into small pieces and use them in stir-fries or toss into bulgur pilaf. (See page 171 for dried dates.)

Figs (Phases 3 & 4)
6.4 g Net Carbs per fresh small fig

Like dates, figs are available both fresh and dried; dried figs can get a whopping 90 percent of their calories from sugar! Look for fresh figs in markets from late spring to late summer. (See page 171 for dried figs.)

Guava (Phases 3 & 4)
5.3 g Net Carbs per ½ cup

When it comes to vitamin C, this tropical fruit is off the charts. You may have trouble finding fresh ones outside of a supermarket with a large Latin clientele.

Loquat (Phases 3 & 4)
14.2 g Net Carbs per 10 loquats

Loquats have an apricot-colored skin, but the fruit tastes more like a plum. Loquats are very fragile and don't ship well, so they're rarely seen outside of Florida, California, and areas with similar climates. If you do find them, choose large ones. They make a tasty addition to a chicken salad.

Lychees (Phases 3 & 4)
14.5 g Net Carbs per ½ cup

If your encounters with lychees don't extend beyond Chinese restaurants, you might not recognize them in supermarkets: These creamy white, sweet fruits come encased in a rough, reddish-brown shell. Look for lychees from June through mid-July.

Pears (Phases 3 & 4)
17.7 g Net Carbs per small Bosc pear;
21.1 g per medium Bartlett

Pears are quite high in sugar, but they supply good amounts of soluble (i.e., cholesterol-lowering) fiber as well as some vitamin C. Leave the peels on, though, to get the most of both nutrients. In addition to the elegant brownish Bosc and red and yellow Bartletts, look for rounded Comice and tiny Seckel or Forelle pears, particularly around the holidays.

Persimmons (Phases 3 & 4)
12.6 g Net Carbs per ½ persimmon

In season from October through February, persimmons are ripe when they are plump, firm, and glossy. They provide some vitamin C, and they also contain alpha carotene, beta carotene, and beta cryptoxanthin.

Pomegranates (Phases 3 & 4)
6.4 g Net Carbs per ¼ pomegranate

Pomegranates' crimson flesh is high in anthocyanins, as well as catechins and ellagic acid. These compounds may make this fruit even higher in antioxidant potency than green tea or red wine. Pomegranates are in season from early fall to early winter, but are at their best around Thanksgiving.

Quince (Phases 3 & 4)
12.3 g Net Carbs per quince

Very astringent and dry in texture, quinces are almost always cooked. Look for them from mid-autumn through late winter.

Rhubarb (Phases 1-4)
1.7 g Net Carbs per ½ cup raw, unsweetened

Unpalatably tart in its raw state, rhubarb is usually cooked with sweetener. Although rhubarb is, botanically, a vegetable, it's most commonly used as a fruit. It becomes sweeter as it's cooked, so add sweetener after it's tender.

SUPER-SIZE FRUIT

You know that food manufacturers can play fast and loose with serving sizes—it's not unusual for a package that looks as though it would serve one to sport a Nutrition Facts label for 2 or 3 servings. Fruit growers and supermarket buyers are attempting to do the same with fruit. Consider this chart, which compares the USDA's definition of a "medium" fruit to the typical size found in a supermarket:

FRUIT	MEDIUM	TYPICAL
Apple (diameter)	2¾ inches	3½ inches
Banana (length)	7–7⅞ inches	9 inches
Cantaloupe (diameter)	5 inches	6 inches
Peach (diameter)	2½ inches	3–3½ inches
Pear	2½ pears	2 pears
Plum (diameter)	2⅛ inches	2½ inches
Strawberry (diameter)	1¼ inches	2–2½ inches

Larger fruits obviously contain more Net Carbs than smaller ones, but there are other reasons to choose small-to-medium-size fruit. Larger fruits often have insipid flavors and woody textures; smaller ones have a truer fruit flavor.

The Deli Counter

Cold cuts and deli meats are convenient to keep on hand, but you need to purchase them carefully. For starters, skip the meats in blister packs sold in the meat department—they tend to have more preservatives; opt for meats from the deli counter, but be choosy.

Steer clear of honey-baked hams and sugar-cured meats, and ask about the ingredients in marinated meats—chicken and turkey may be basted with a sauce that contains added sugars. Also, seek out "house-made" and "house-roasted" beef, pork, and turkey breast. These are almost always made by roasting the actual cut of meat, not made of processed meat and fillers, such as bread crumbs, animal parts, and flavor enhancers like MSG.

Watch out for cold cuts and any smoked and cured meats, too. These can be high in nitrates, which the body converts to nitrites—and they are potential carcinogens, if consumed regularly and in excess. Small amounts are unlikely to be harmful, but seek out alternatives whenever possible.

Always use caution when selecting prepared salads. Potato, rice, and pasta salads will of course be too high in carbohydrates, but even salads you might think are acceptable, such as tuna, tomato and cucumber salads, as well as white fish salad and coleslaw, can contain hidden carbs. Request a list of ingredients at the deli counter to be sure you're not getting too many carbs. And skip such classic deli items as knishes, noodle pudding and rice pudding—all are high in carbs and lack much nutritional value.

For information on cheeses, see page 112.

➤ COLD CUTS ◄

Bologna, Beef (Phases 1-4)
4.0 g Net Carbs per 3½ ounces

Chicken Breast Roll, Roasted (Phases 1-4)
1.8 g Net Carbs per 3½ ounces

⚠ **Chopped Liver**
2 g Net Carbs per ¼ cup
  Contains trans fats and added sugars.

Ham, Extra-Lean (Phases 1-4)
1 g Net Carbs per 3½ ounces

⚠ **Ham, Honey, Smoked**
7.2 g Net Carbs per 3½ ounces
  Contains added sugars.

Ham, Regular (not lean) (Phases 1-4)
2.5 g Net Carbs per 3½ ounces

⚠ **Liverwurst**
0.9 g Net Carbs per 3½ ounces
  May contain added sugars.

Pastrami (Phases 1-4)
3.1 g Net Carbs per 3½ ounces

Prosciutto (Phases 1-4)
5 g Net Carbs per 3½ ounces

Salami, Italian (Phases 1-4)
1.2 g Net Carbs per 3½ ounces

Turkey Breast, Roasted (Phases 1-4)
0 g Net Carbs per 6 ounces

**Turkey Breast, Smoked, Lemon-Pepper Flavor
(Phases 1-4)**
1.3 g Net Carbs per 3½ ounces

Turkey Ham (Phases 1-4)
1.5 g Net Carbs per 3½ ounces

> **WORST BITES:** Asian-Style Prepared Foods
> Although some produce is high in Net Carbs,
> most of it has some nutritional value. Not so with the
> prepared foods, particularly wonton skins, egg roll
> wrappers, and Chinese noodles. With 32–41 grams of
> Net Carbs per serving—and with controlled-carb tor-
> tillas and pastas available to use instead—you'll have
> plenty of alternatives for avoiding these.

---

10 DELICIOUS MEAL SHORTCUTS
FROM THE DELI

Craving something that tastes like a home-cooked meal but
doesn't require the time or the fuss? Need a fast yet elegant
hors d'oeuvre? These ten shortcuts using items found at the
deli can help:

1. **Spicy beef-wrapped asparagus:** Slather thinly
   sliced roast beef with a blend of horseradish and
   mayo, then wrap around two lightly steamed asparagus spears. (Phases1-4; 2 g Net Carbs)
2. **Italian ham roll-ups:** Spread thinly sliced prosciutto with a tablespoon of garlicky hummus or a mixture
   of pesto and mayonnaise; roll up.
   (Phases 2-4; 2 g Net Carbs)

3. **Speedy navy bean soup:** Get ½ pound of ham sliced as thickly as possible (ideally ¼-inch or thicker). Cut into cubes. Heat water with a chicken bouillon cube, then add ham and ½ cup organic, no-salt-added canned navy beans. Let simmer for 20 minutes. (Phases 3 & 4; 11 g Net Carbs)

4. **Almost-instant chicken noodle soup:** Break 2 ounces of Atkins Quick Quisine Pasta Cuts spaghetti into 2–4-inch lengths; cook in boiling chicken broth, made with water and a chicken bouillon cube. Meanwhile, pull the meat off of a rotisserie chicken. Add to the soup and heat through.
(Phases 2-4; 6 g Net Carbs)

5. **Almost-instant Italian-inspired soup:** Combine 2 tablespoons tomato purée with chicken broth made from water and a chicken bouillon cube. Add coarsely chopped salami, 2 ounces cubed mozzarella and a handful of slivered basil. Heat to serving temperature. (Phases 1–4; 3 g Net Carbs)

6. **Chicken quesadillas:** Buy grilled chicken cutlets at the deli. Cut them into strips. Set an Atkins Bakery Tortilla on a baking sheet. Sprinkle grated cheese over half of the tortilla, arrange chicken strips on cheese, then sprinkle chicken with more cheese. Fold the tortilla over the cheese and press closed. Bake in a 350°F oven until the cheese melts, then cut into three wedges. (Phases 2-4; 5 g Net Carbs)

7. **Zesty beef salad:** Cut thinly sliced deli roast beef into strips. Toss with ½ cup mixed salad greens, a handful of mint and cilantro leaves, and your favorite controlled-carb dressing. (Phases 1-4; 2 g Net Carbs)

8. **Grilled chicken tossed salad:** Combine a sliced, grilled chicken cutlet, ½ cup mixed salad greens, 2 tablespoons of crumbled blue cheese, and 2 tablespoons sliced almonds, toasted; toss with your favorite controlled-carb salad dressing.
(Phases 2-4; 3 g Net Carbs)

9. **Creamy curry chicken salad:** Remove the skin from a rotisserie chicken; pull the meat off the bone and shred. In a large bowl, combine mayonnaise, curry powder, and thinly sliced scallion. Add the chicken and ¼ cup of sliced water chestnuts. (Phases 2-4; 4 g Net Carbs)

10. **Easy pizzas:** Pick up some meatballs (be sure they contain no bread crumbs), roasted peppers or antipasto, and Genoa salami or pepperoni. Set an Atkins Bakery Tortilla on a baking sheet, sprinkle lightly with cheese. Spread with tomato paste, then top with your choice of sliced meatballs or sausage, veggies, sliced black olives, chopped garlic, or other toppings. (Phases 2-4; 7 g Net Carbs)

➤ SAUSAGE, LUNCH MEATS, ◄ AND CURED MEATS

Sausages can be fresh, dried, cooked, or smoked. Cured meats can be smoked, brined, pickled, or salted. Both can be either mild or highly seasoned.

Sausages are made by grinding meats, combining them with fat, spices or seasonings, and possibly fillers, such as bread crumbs, cereals, soybean flour and dried-milk solids, used to stretch the meat; then the mixture is typically stuffed into casings. Given the range of possible fillers, it's easy to see how sausages can be concealing added carbohydrates—be sure to read ingredients labels carefully and avoid sausages containing unacceptable ingredients.

Choose cured meats carefully. Curing extends storage life and is typically done using salt and/or smoke. However, if sugar is used in the curing liquid, some of it may penetrate the meat and add carbohydrates. In addition, nitrates are frequently used in the process of curing (they impart a pinkish-red color to foods like ham and bacon). Seek out fresh sausages, which are nitrate free, and nitrate-free bacon and other meats (you may have to ask at the meat counter, or go to a specialty butcher). Applegate Farms is one brand offering nitrate-free meats.

As with cuts of meat, it isn't necessary to weigh portions, but it's wise to pay attention to portion size. For example, if you've cooked a pound of kielbasa, cutting it into eight pieces will give you 2-ounce servings. Because brands of these meats can vary regionally, we've provided average Net Carb information rather than brand-specific data.

Italian Sausage, Pork (Phases 1-4)
0.9 g Net Carbs per 2 ounces
This fresh sausage comes sweet or hot, and sweet simply means "not spicy," rather than sweetened. Links are most common, but you may find sausage patties or bulk sausage.

Pork Sausage (Phases 1-4)
1 g Net Carbs per link or patty
Like Italian sausage, breakfast sausage is seasoned and often includes high-carb fillers, like bread crumbs, oatmeal or flours. It can be formed into links or patties, and may be sold bulk as well.

Kielbasa (Phases 1-4)
0.8 g Net Carbs per 2 ounces
Available made with pork, beef, turkey, or a blend of all three, kielbasa can vary widely in fat content (turkey is the leanest). For best flavor, choose beef, pork, or a blend.

Smoked Sausage (Phases 1-4)
- **Sweet** *3 g Net Carbs per link*
- **Beef** *1 g Net Carbs per link*
- **Hot** *2 g Net Carbs per link*

As with Italian sausages, smoked sausages are available sweet or hot. Because they are heat-and-serve, you're more likely to find them near hams and kielbasa rather than with the fresh meats.

Knockwurst (Phases 1-4)
2.3 g Net Carbs per link

Bratwurst (Phases 1-4)
2.1 g Net Carbs per link

Beef Hot Dogs (Phases 1-4)
1.2 g Net Carbs per hot dog

Beef-Pork Hot Dogs (Phases 1-4)
1.5 g Net Carbs per hot dog

Cheddarwurst (Phases 1-4)
2 g Net Carbs per link

Cheese Dogs (Phases 1-4)
1.3 g Net Carbs per link
Even if you skip the bun and sweetened condiments, you still may be surprised at the carb content of these sausages; they frequently contain cereals as filler. Skip the typical fixings—instead, slice the franks or wursts, pan-fry them, and add them to a veggie soup or controlled-carb mac and cheese.

Andouille Sausage (Phases 1-4)
1 g Net Carbs per 2 ounces
A French sausage made from pork chitterlings and tripe, andouille is smoked and very spicy. It's a key ingredient in gumbo and jambalaya.

Chorizo Sausage (Phases 1-4)
1 g Net Carbs per 2 ounces (or 1 4-inch link)

Linguiça Sausage (Phases 1-4)
1 g Net Carbs per 2 ounces

Popular in Portuguese, Spanish, and Latin cooking, these spicy, garlicky sausages are a terrific way to add flavor to soups and vegetable dishes. Both sausages are deep red and look like other, fully cooked sausages, but both chorizo and linguiça are fresh and need to be cooked thoroughly.

Flavored Sausage (Phases 2-4)
0-2 g Net Carbs per 2.5 ounces
In varieties like chicken apple, roasted garlic and sundried tomato, these flavored sausages contain dehydrated fruits and other carb-containing ingredients, so they are not acceptable during Induction.

Bacon (Phases 1-4)
0.1 g Net Carbs per 3 slices

Canadian Bacon (Phases 1-4)
0.9 g Net Carbs per 3 slices

Pancetta (Phases 1-4)
0.2 g Net Carbs per ounce
Though pancetta is sometimes referred to as Italian bacon, it isn't smoked the way American bacon is; it's just cured with a mixture of seasonings. Canadian bacon is actually closer to ham—it's smoked, not cured, so it's already cooked, and it comes from the loin rather than the belly.

Prosciutto (Phases 1-4)
0.9 g Net Carbs per 6 ounces

Ham, luncheon meat (Phases 1-4)
1.8 g Net Carbs per 6 ounces

Ham, boneless, canned or in plastic (Phases 1-4)
0 g Net Carbs
Luncheon meat hams and the sort that come in cryovac (the heavy, heat-sealed plastic) and cans are more accurately

called "ham and water products"—they are injected with a
brine that cures them much more rapidly than dry-cured
hams like country ham or prosciutto, the famous Italian ham.

Beef Bologna (Phases 1-4)
2.0 g Net Carbs per 3 slices

Beef-Pork Bologna (Phases 1-4)
2.4 g Net Carbs per 3 slices

Beef Salami (Phases 1-4)
1.9 g Net Carbs per 3 slices

Beef-Pork Salami (Phases 1-4)
0.8 g Net Carbs per 3 slices

Pork Salami (Phases 1-4)
0.5 g Net Carbs per 3 slices

Pepperoni (Phases 1-4)
0.8 g Net Carbs per 5 pieces

Pastrami (Phases 1-4)
5.2 g Net Carbs per 6 ounces

Pork Roll (Phases 1-4)
0.3 g Net Carbs per 3 ounces

⚠ Liverwurst
2 g Net Carbs per 2 ounces
  May contain added sugars.

FYI Olive Loaf (Phases 3 & 4)
7.8 g Net Carbs per 3 slices
  Contains filler.

FYI Scrapple (Phases 3 & 4)
7.9 g Net Carbs per 2 ounces
  Contains filler.

Nearly all of these meats contain nitrates; not all of them are available in a nitrate-free form. Several of them are fairly high in Net Carbs as well. You're best off consuming these in small portions, if at all. Rather than buy blister-packs of pre-sliced luncheon meats, stop at the deli for fresher meats with better flavor.

➤ PRESEASONED AND ◄ HEAT-AND-SERVE MEATS

If you're pressed for time, you may well be tempted to pick up seasoned pork tenderloins, heat-and-serve meatloaf, or brasciole (meat rolled around cheese and greens). Few of these are wise choices for controlled-carb meals.

Flavor, quality, and carbohydrate content vary by brand, and although some brands are available nationally, others are regional. If you opt for shortcut entrees, start by seeking out flavorings that don't sound sweetened—lemon pepper will probably be lower in Net Carbs than teriyaki or honey glazed, for example.

PRESEASONED MEATS

Pork Brasciole (Phases 1-4)
2 g Net Carbs per 2.5 ounces

Beef or Lamb Kebabs (Phases 1-4)
1 g Net Carbs per kebab

Items such as these are usually made in-store, and although they seldom contain Nutrition Facts labels they may list ingredients (or you may be able to ask at the meat counter what goes into them). Brasciole, or pinwheels, will contain some Net Carbs from cheese, and the kebabs will as well, depending on which vegetables are included. If you're craving stuffed pork chops, you'll be better off buying thick chops and making your own stuffing for them. Ditto with pork tenderloins. Season them with herbs and spices or controlled-carb marinades, like Atkins Quick Quisine Teriyaki Sauce.

Pork Tenderloin (Phases 1-4)
- **Peppercorn** *2g Net Carbs per 4 ounces*
- **Lemon Garlic** *2 g Net Carbs per 4 ounces*
- **Garden Herb** *3 g Net Carbs per 4 ounces*
- ⚠ **Teriyaki** *5.2 g Net Carbs per 4 ounces*
  Contains added sugars.

HEAT-AND-EAT ENTREES

Packaged entrees with noodles or rice in the mix are as high in Net Carbs as you might imagine, but nearly all of them contain more Net Carbs than is reasonable—gravies are almost invariably thickened with cornstarch or modified potato starch. Choose these wisely, examining ingredients lists with a fine-tooth comb, and reserve them for nights when you're most pressed for time.

Italian Seasoned Pork Roast (Phases 2-4)
4 g Net Carbs per 5 ounces

Beef Steak Dinner (Phases 2-4)
3 g Net Carbs per 5 ounces

⚠ **Meatloaf in Tomato Sauce**
9 g Net Carbs per 5 ounces
  Contains added sugars.

FYI **Beef with Gravy (Phases 3 & 4)**
4 g Net Carbs per 5 ounces
  Contains flour.

⚠ **Glazed Ham**
7 g Net Carbs per 5 ounces
  Contains added sugars.

WORST BITES: If you need a fast fix for supper, consider your options carefully. Unseasoned meat is completely free of carbohydrate. From there, uncooked seasoned and prepared meat entrees are your next best bet. Heat-and-serve entrees are even riskier—some are acceptable, but others qualify as Worst Bites, particularly if you consider the numbers at a realistic portion size, rather than what the package label says.

- **Pork barbecue**   *12 g Net Carbs per ¼ cup*
- **Beef barbecue**   *12 g Net Carbs per ¼ cup*
- **Corndogs**   *15 g Net Carbs per corndog*
- **Stuffed pork chops** *15 g Net Carbs per chop*
- **Breaded veal patties** *16 g Net Carbs per patty*
- **Breaded beef patties** *16 g Net Carbs per patty*
- **Beef roast**   *18 g Net Carbs per 5 ounces*
- **Taquitos**   *24 g Net Carbs per taquito*
- **Beef burritos**   *33 g Net Carbs per burrito*
- **Beef and bean chimichangas**   *33 g Net Carbs per chimichanga*

The Fish Counter

Fish, particularly cold-water fish, provides a host of nutritional benefits. Fish is an excellent source of omega-3 fatty acids, a type of polyunsaturated fat that is essential to proper cell function and has been linked to cardiovascular health. Most fish are high in protein and B vitamins (particularly B_{12}), minerals like zinc and selenium, and they provide varying degrees of vitamins A, D, and E. Fish, with the exception of shellfish, contains no carbohydrate.

If you've bought into the rumor that fish is difficult to cook, give it a chance. Most do cook rapidly and can go from tender to rubbery in a flash, but unless you're roasting a whole fish or lobster, most finfish and shellfish recipes can be on the table in about 30 minutes. Find great-tasting, easy fish and seafood recipes at *www.atkins.com*.

➤ FRESH FISH ◄

Fish can be categorized in a variety of ways, but for nutritional and culinary purposes, warm-water (or lean) and cold-water (or fatty) are more important than freshwater and saltwater, or round fish and flatfish. Warm-water fish typically has white flesh and is exceptionally low in fat. Cold-water fish tends to have darker flesh and contain more than 5 percent heart-healthy fat by weight.

WARM-WATER FISH

Most warm-water, or lean, fish have a mild, slightly sweet flavor and a fine flake, though some (cod, for example) flake in large chunks. They are interchangeable in most recipes. You may find more exotic species in your market depending on seasonality and availability, but these are the most common and readily available. A standard portion of fish is about 6 ounces uncooked.

Bass (Phases 1-4)
0 g Net Carbs

Look for firm flesh; its color can range from white to a pearly beige-pink, but it should be translucent. Bass has a mild, sweet flavor and is quite flaky.

Catfish (Phases 1-4)
0 g Net Carbs

Fillets are white to pale pink, and may have yellow stripes on them. Catfish has a large flake.

Cod (Phases 1-4)
0 g Net Carbs

The cod family includes scrod, hake, pollack, and haddock. Cod flakes easily into large pieces. Salt cod, sometimes called bacalao, which must be soaked in water before being cooked, is also carb-free.

Flounder (Phases 1-4)
0 g Net Carbs

Like its close cousin sole, flounder is a flat fish with a very fine flake, pearly gray flesh, and sweet, mild flavor.

Halibut (Phases 1-4)
0 g Net Carbs

Whether your market sells halibut in steaks or fillets, look for firm, pearly white flesh; those that are less than 1 inch thick will be more tender.

Monkfish (Phases 1-4)
0 g Net Carbs

Monkfish's texture is reminiscent of sea scallops or lobster, and its flavor is mild and slightly sweet. Its flesh should be creamy white.

Perch (Phases 1-4)
0 g Net Carbs

Whether you buy freshwater or ocean perch, look for white to beige-pink flesh with a firm, close-grained texture.

Snapper (Phases 1-4)
0 g Net Carbs

True, red snapper is a rarity at supermarket counters, and the real deal is quite pricey. (Often, Pacific perch is marketed as snapper.) Red snapper has a pearly pink flesh and a deep reddish-orange skin, and if the fish is whole, you'll know it's authentic snapper by its red eyes.

Tilapia (Phases 1-4)
0 g Net Carbs

Tilapia has a white-to-pink flesh and somewhat soft texture. Almost all tilapia sold is farm-raised.

COLD-WATER FISH

Fish that live in cold water have larger amounts of fat than those that inhabit warmer water. Their greater distribution of fat makes them generally firmer in texture and meatier. Cold-water fish is one of the few foods that is high in omega-3 fatty acids (flaxseed, walnuts and canola oil are others). These essential fats can protect against heart disease and high blood pressure, and can reduce levels of triglycerides as well as improve autoimmune diseases like lupus and rheumatoid arthritis. Although many of these fish are similar in flavor or texture, some are quite distinctive.

FISH: FRESH VS. FROZEN

When it comes to fish, frozen isn't necessarily bad—in fact, it's often preferable to fresh. Deep-sea fish like swordfish and tuna is almost always frozen at sea, since fishing boats can remain at sea for several weeks; freezing prevents them from spoiling. Shrimp, scallops, and lobster are often frozen at sea, too. Sometimes, but not always, it's thawed by the time you buy it.

If you plan to freeze your fish when you get it home, ask the counterperson if the fish has been thawed. The store may have frozen fish in the back that you can buy instead. It's safer not to freeze any food more than once.

Most markets have a freezer section by the fish department. Though it's often stocked with high-carb, heat-and-serve foods, look there for individually quick-frozen fillets. If properly handled, these can be very high quality. They're often packed in opaque bags so you won't be able to see whether the fish has ice crystals, but press it in a few places. If you feel crushed ice or if some of the fish feels mushy, pass on it.

Fish spoils quickly. If you're buying fresh (or thawed) fish, skip those on styrofoam trays in plastic wrap. These can go bad more rapidly than fish that's wrapped for you. If the pre-wrapped fish is your only alternative, smell it. Spoilage will be obvious, even through the plastic.

The best indicator of freshness is the eyes, and if you're buying whole fish, check to see that the eyes aren't sunken or cloudy. The second best sign is texture: The flesh should feel firm when pressed. Of course you can't poke it to see how resilient it is, but ask the counterperson to do it—and watch closely to see if the flesh springs back quickly. If the fillets pass this test, ask to smell them. Don't be shy about this request: You're paying for it, and fish is comparatively expensive.

Anchovies (Phases 1-4)
0 g Net Carbs
It's unlikely you'll find fresh anchovies in a supermarket, but if you do, be sure they are on ice—anchovies can go bad quickly. Anchovies are an excellent source of omega-3s.

Bluefish (Phases 1-4)
0 g Net Carbs
Fresh bluefish has a blue-gray flesh and steely blue skin. Older, less fresh bluefish has a strong, oily flavor. They're a good source of omega-3s.

Mackerel (Phases 1-4)
0 g Net Carbs
Often sold whole, these small fish are sometimes sold as fillets. Look for bright, almost vividly colored skin. Mackerel is a wonderfully rich source of omega-3s.

Mahi Mahi (dolphin fish) (Phases 1-4)
0 g Net Carbs
Mahi mahi is completely unrelated to dolphin—it's a fish, not a mammal. It has a mild, sweet flavor and its flesh can be beige to rose-colored and should be quite firm. Mahi mahi is fairly low in omega-3s.

Salmon (Phases 1-4)
0 g Net Carbs
There are six major types of salmon: pink, chum, sockeye, coho, king (sometimes called Chinook), and Atlantic. Each type of salmon has a different nutrient composition, and the levels of nutrients can fluctuate throughout the year. Salmon is high in omega-3s.

Sardines (Phases 1-4)
0 g Net Carbs
As with anchovies, fresh sardines are a rarity in most supermarkets. Fresh sardines taste remarkably different from

canned ones, so if you find them, try them split and grilled. Sardines are exceptionally rich in omega-3s.

Shark (Phases 1-4)
0 g Net Carbs

Most shark is from mako or blacktip; shark should be white to pink in color with a firm, resilient flesh. Its flavor is somewhat milder than swordfish. Shark provides moderate amounts of omega-3s.

Swordfish (Phases 1-4)
0 g Net Carbs

Fresh swordfish has a pearly, glistening sheen to it; its color indicates the fish's diet, not its quality (shrimp turns it a pinkish hue). Swordfish contains moderate levels of omega-3s.

Trout (Phases 1-4)
0 g Net Carbs

Fish from this huge family can be palest pink or deep orange. Whether you find freshwater trout like rainbow or brook or sea-going trout like steelhead, trout should have a firm, fine-grained flesh. Most trout are moderately high in omega-3s.

Tuna (Phases 1-4)
0 g Net Carbs

Tuna steaks range in color from pale pink (albacore) to ruby red (yellowfin) to almost maroon (big eye); darker tuna tends to be more robustly flavored. Albacore is lower in omega-3s than other varieties.

FACTS ABOUT FARM-RAISED FISH

If you've noticed a bigger variety at your market's fish counter, you're seeing the effects of aquaculture, or fish farming.

Aquaculture helps to stabilize the fish market. It reduces fluctuations in availability and price of the fish, and because farm-raised fish is fed a specific diet, aquaculture helps to ensure consistency in flavor and appearance, too.

Detractors, however, believe that farm-raised fish tastes blander than wild fish. Because farm-raised fish lives in pens or tanks, it may be fed antibiotics to reduce disease. Some fish farmers are seeking approval to use growth hormones, which would get the fish to market sooner.

That isn't to say that all wild fish is good for you. PCBs and mercury can build up in fish over time, so large, long-lived predatory fish like tuna, swordfish, and shark can harbor higher levels of these and other toxins. The Environmental Protection Agency closely monitors fisheries for pesticides and metals and ensures that these farm-raised fish are safe.

Your best bet is to eat an array of fish from a variety of sources. If your diet includes freshwater and saltwater fish, large and small, lean and fatty, finned and shellfish, you'll lessen your exposure to harmful elements while obtaining a variety of nutrients. You should also limit consumption of fish to no more than 12 ounces per week, which is especially important if you're pregnant or nursing.

➤ FRESH SHELLFISH ◄

Long reviled because of its high cholesterol content, shellfish is actually fine for most people to eat—very few people experience a rise in blood cholesterol levels from eating foods that are high in cholesterol. It is actually your own liver that produces most of the cholesterol in your blood.

Shellfish is incredibly perishable and should only be purchased on the day you plan to cook it (or buy frozen shellfish and put it in the freezer as soon as you get home). Some shellfish is purchased live—lobster, clams, and mussels, for example. Choose feisty lobsters and tightly closed bivalves, and if they're packed in plastic at the store, remove them when you get home so they don't suffocate.

Smell shellfish to be sure it has a briny aroma and avoid anything that smells musty or like ammonia. If you have any doubts about the shellfish, ask to see the tags that certify the shellfish came from unpolluted beds. (By law, fishmongers are required to keep these tags.)

Also, keep in mind that clams, oysters and mussels are higher in carbs than other shellfish, so limit your portion size to 4 ounces without shells. Squid and scallops aren't that much lower.

Clams, cooked (Phases 1-4)
8 g Net Carbs per 6 ounces

Hard-shelled clams include littlenecks and cherrystones. Soft-shells are sometimes called steamers. Hard-shelled clams should be tightly closed; soft-shelled ones partly opened. Avoid either with cracked or broken shells.

Crabmeat, cooked (Phases 1-4)
0 g Net Carbs per 6 ounces

With the exception of soft-shell crabs, most crabmeat is sold already cooked. Still, it's extremely perishable. It's usually sold in tubs, and you should ask the counter person to open the tub so you can smell it. It should smell of the ocean. (Canned and pasteurized refrigerated crabmeat is not as perishable.) Beware of imitation crab legs, or surimi, which is made from pollock or whiting and often contains fillers such as potatoes.

Lobster, steamed (Phases 1-4)
6 g Net Carbs per pound

Live lobster should be very active—watch closely as it's

lifted from the tank to be sure it's waving its claws and flapping its tail.

Mussels, steamed (Phases 1-4)
8.4 g Net Carbs per 4 ounces

Look for tightly closed mussel shells; if they are loose, choose ones that feel only moderately heavy (really heavy ones may be full of sand). Mussel meat is also available in tubs; these mussels should be plump and juicy looking, and beige to orange in color. Mussels provide some omega-3s.

Oysters, raw (Phases 1-4)
4.5 g Net Carbs per 4 ounces

Oyster shells should be tightly closed or should snap shut if tapped. Shucked meat should be beige and the broth it's in should be only slightly cloudy. Oysters provide some omega-3s.

Scallops, raw (Phases 1-4)
4 g Net Carbs per 6 ounces

Whether you choose sea scallops (up to 1½ inches in diameter), bay scallops (about ¾ inch) or calicos (up to ½ inch), scallops should be firm, with a translucent flesh. Bay and sea scallops are sweeter than calicos.

Shrimp, cooked (Phases 1-4)
0 g Net Carbs per 6 ounces

Ignore signs about the number of shrimp to a pound—what's considered "extra-large" at one market may be "medium" at another. Instead, purchase shrimp by the pound, and don't forget that there's considerable waste with the shells. (Figure at least 1½–2 pounds for four.) Shrimp should look firm and should fill the shells.

Squid, raw (Phases 1-4)
6 g Net Carbs per 6 ounces

Choose calamari with small (no longer than 4 inches), milky white bodies and maroon tentacles; larger ones tend to be tough.

➤ **PREPARED FISH AND SHELLFISH** ◄

Most stores sell prepared fish and shellfish behind the counter, or in a refrigerator or freezer case near the fish counter.

Sometimes, these are prepared at the store, and you should be able to find out what ingredients are included by asking someone in the store's fish department. If you get a vague answer, play it safe—skip the prepared fish and make your own.

Fish and shellfish from the refrigerator and freezer cases can vary considerably among brands. In general, though, fish cakes, breaded and battered fillets, and stuffed shellfish are high in carbohydrate. Pickled herring may contain sugar or another sweetener, and some salmon is coated with a sugar mixture before smoking and curing, so read the list of ingredients when one is provided. Watch out for seafood salads, which may contain hidden carbs or sweeteners.

Pickled Herring, boneless (Phases 1-4)
2 g Net Carbs per ounce

Lox/Smoked Salmon (Phases 1-4)
0 g Net Carbs per 6 ounces

Salt Cod (Bacalao) (Phases 1-4)
0 g Net Carbs per 3 ounces

Mussels, in Tomato Sauce (Phases 2-4)
7.2 g Net Carbs per 15 mussels

Shrimp Scampi (Phases 1-4)
5 g Net Carbs per 4 ounces (8-10 shrimp)

Whitefish Salad (Phases 1-4)
0 g Net Carbs per cup

FYI Clams Casino (Phases 3 & 4)
7 g Net Carbs per 2 clams
   Contains bread crumbs.

FYI Clams Oreganato (Phases 3 & 4)
6 g Net Carbs per 2 clams
   Contains bread crumbs.

WORST BITES: You know that convenience
foods are more expensive, but here's proof that
you pay twice—the second time in astronomical carb
counts. It takes about two minutes to bread flounder or
shrimp and five minutes to whip up crab cakes or fish
cakes, so these prepared foods aren't huge timesavers.
And when you make them yourself, you can use Atkins
Quick Quisine Bake Mix or another controlled-carb
breading.

   Pass on self-serve soups kept warm in large kettles
in the seafood department, too. While you can prepare
cream-based soups, like lobster bisque and New
England clam chowder, at home without high-carb ingredients, these versions will no doubt contain potatoes or other starchy vegetables or bleached white
flour, and because they bear no ingredients label, it's
impossible to know how much.

- **Crab delights, surimi**   *10 g Net Carbs per ½ cup*
- **Imitation crabmeat**   *10 g Net Carbs per ½ cup*
- **Stuffed clams**   *16 g Net Carbs per clam*
- **Crab cakes**   *18 g Net Carbs per cake*
- **Breaded flounder**   *20 g Net Carbs per 3.5*
  ounces
- **Breaded shrimp**   *22 g Net Carbs per 7*
  shrimp
- **Sweet & sour shrimp**   *28 g Net Carbs per 6*
  shrimp
- **Fish cakes**   *29 g Net Carbs per 2 cakes*

The Meat Department

Meat—whether beef, pork, lamb, or veal—supplies protein, fat, B vitamins, and iron, but absolutely no carbohydrate. It's only when you get into the cured and prepared meat products that you need to pay careful attention to ensure you're not getting unpleasant surprises.

Although you don't need to worry about weighing foods or counting calories when you're doing Atkins, it's still wise to pay attention to portion sizes. If you fill up on a large steak, for instance, you may be too full to have your vegetables, meaning that you don't get enough other nutrients. Plus, eating huge portions of protein can cause the body to convert some of it to blood glucose, which will hinder a fat-burning metabolism. Start with about eight ounces of raw meat per person—that is, buy 2 pounds of boneless meat to serve four.

You'll also want to limit portions of meat products that do include carbohydrates, as well as cured meats. Bacon, ham, hot dogs, and the like are made with nitrates in order to preserve freshness. These compounds are harmless outside of the body, but when you eat them they convert to nitrites, which have been proven to be carcinogens when consumed over time.

➤ BEEF ◄

High in protein, iron, and vitamin B_{12}, beef is available in almost endless variety, from quick-to-cook tender steaks to tougher cuts that require long, slow cooking. Sometimes, cuts go by different names in different parts of the country; here are commonly available cuts:

Ground (Phases 1-4)
0 g Net Carbs

Ground beef is quite versatile. Form it into a juicy burger, or use it to make meatballs, add it to chili and tomato sauce, or brown it for the base of a simple stir-fry.

Short Loin Cuts (Phases 1-4)
0 g Net Carbs

The short loin is the middle of the animal's back. These cuts are often quite tender because this area gets so little exercise, and they are quite expensive as well. They are best cooked with dry heat—grilled, roasted, pan-seared, or broiled.

Quick-cooking cuts: Steaks such as filet mignon, top loin, T-bone, porterhouse, strip loin, bone-in top loin, shell steak, strip steak, Delmonico, club steak, Kansas City steaks, New York strip steaks, and boneless club steaks.

Longer-cooking cuts: Whole tenderloin.

Rib Cuts (Phases 1-4)
0 g Net Carbs

Muscles by the rib get more exercise than the short loin, so rib cuts tend to be slightly less tender than short loin steaks, but some believe they are higher in flavor.

Quick-cooking cuts: Steaks such as rib-eye and rib steaks.
Longer-cooking cuts: Prime rib.

Sirloin Cuts (Phases 1-4)
0 g Net Carbs

Sirloin cuts come from the lower back; like rib cuts, they're less tender but higher in flavor than short loin cuts. Because sirloin steaks are leaner than rib steaks, they are better marinated. This area is composed of many muscles that can be cut in a variety of ways.

Quick-cooking cuts: Steaks such as tri-tip, top butt, top sirloin, sirloin butt, hip sirloin, center-cut sirloin, and London broil.

Longer-cooking cuts: Triangle roast, sirloin roast, sirloin tip roast, and ball tip roast.

Round Cuts (Phases 1-4)
0 g Net Carbs

Round cuts are those from the hip or hindquarters. Because muscles in this area get frequent use, they tend to be tough. Marinate steaks or cut them into strips for a stir-fry; roasts should be braised or pot-roasted.

Quick-cooking cuts: Steaks such as London broil, top round, or round tip.

Longer-cooking cuts: Bottom round, round steak, top round, rump roast, and eye of the round.

Flank Steaks (Phases 1-4)
0 g Net Carbs

Cut from the chest and sides, flank steak, hanger steak, and skirt steak are somewhat chewy but very flavorful. Originally, London broil was cut from the flank, but because this is a fairly small area and the steak became so popular, butchers began cutting it from other areas. Flank cuts should be marinated, then grilled or broiled and sliced across the grain. They're also delicious cubed for shish kebabs.

Chuck Cuts (Phases 1-4)
0 g Net Carbs

The chuck includes the shoulder—areas that get considerable exercise. Although you might find chuck steaks, you're more likely to find chuck sold as blade, arm roast, chuck eye, or cross-rib roast. All cuts from the chuck are better braised.

Brisket (Phases 1-4)
0 g Net Carbs

The upper portion of the forelegs and the area between them gets considerable exercise and can be quite tough. Sold as brisket, brisket first cut, and brisket front cut, this is always braised or pot-roasted.

➤ PORK ◄

Pork today is much leaner than it was 20 or 30 years ago, so you must choose carefully to be sure you'll get meat that will be flavorful and juicy, rather than tough and dry. Avoid meat that is pale pink or gray, and reach for reddish-pink cuts instead. Pork should feel firm, not soft (press or squeeze it through the plastic wrap).

Unlike beef, most pork is so tender it doesn't need to be braised or pot-roasted to become tender, but some cuts of pork can be braised or stewed with delicious results.

Loin Cuts (Phases 1-4)
0 g Net Carbs
From the pig's back, loin cuts are described as blade loin if they come from near the shoulder, sirloin if they come from near the leg, and center cut; the last tends to be more expensive.

Quick-cooking cuts: Loin chops (these look like pork T-bones), rib chops (bone-in or boneless), sirloin chops, blade chops, tenderloin.

Longer-cooking cuts: Center-cut pork loin (bone-in or boneless), boneless pork loin, blade end pork loin roast, crown roast, tenderloin, baby back ribs, country-style ribs.

Ham (Phases 1-4)
0 g Net Carbs
Although hams are most often cured or smoked, you'll also find fresh hams in supermarkets. Sometimes, cuts from the front leg have butt or ham in their names, which adds to the confusion. Fresh hams are from the hind leg,

not the front, and may be called pork leg, leg of pork, or fresh ham.

Quick-cooking cuts: Pork scallop, fresh ham steak.

Longer-cooking cuts: Whole fresh leg of pork, top leg, fresh ham (shank portion or butt), sirloin pork roast.

Belly Cuts (Phases 1-4)
0 g Net Carbs

Cuts from the belly include spareribs and bacon (see page 73 for bacon), which have wonderful flavor. Cut down on Net Carbs by rubbing pork ribs with a dry spice rub rather than slathering on a sugary sauce.

Shoulder Cuts (Phases 1-4)
0 g Net Carbs

The front leg area of a pig is called the shoulder, but cuts from this area are called the Boston butt or Boston shoulder roast (from the top of the shoulder); cuts from the leg itself are called picnic roasts or picnic hams.

Quick-cooking cuts: Blade chops, country-style rib chops, pork blade steaks.

Longer-cooking cuts: Boston butt, pork shoulder butt, pork butt, arm roast, picnic shoulder roast.

➤ LAMB ◄

The average American eats only about a pound of lamb per year. Lamb can be expensive, but it has a slightly gamy, slightly sweet flavor that marries perfectly with strong seasonings like garlic, lemon, mint, rosemary, and mustard, as well as spices and dried fruits common to Indian and Moroccan cooking.

Lamb is high in iron, protein, zinc, and several of the B vitamins. Choose reddish-pink cuts with pearly white fat; dark red or purple meat and yellow fat are signs of older animals.

Shoulder Cuts (Phases 1-4)
0 g Net Carbs

These muscles get frequent work on a lamb, so they're typically tough; tenderness often depends on how they are cut. Shoulder chops are best braised (brown them first). Cut the larger roasts up for kebabs or stews.

Quick-cooking cuts: Shoulder chops, shoulder arm chops, shoulder blade chops.

Longer-cooking cuts: Square-cut shoulder roast (boneless), lamb shoulder roast (same cut, just rolled and tied).

Rib Cuts (Phases 1-4)
0 g Net Carbs

The back just behind the shoulder, lamb rib is exquisitely tender and delicious. Rib can be left whole or cut into chops.

Quick-cooking cuts: Rib chops.

Longer-cooking cuts: Rack of lamb (this is sometimes Frenched, which means that part of the bones are cleaned of fat and tissue).

Loin Cuts (Phases 1-4)
0 g Net Carbs

The part of the back just above the hip, lamb loin is also quite tender. Lamb tenderloins are quite small (they rarely weigh more than 8 ounces or so) and, unlike beef and pork tenderloins, shouldn't be roasted—broil, grill, or sauté them instead.

Quick-cooking cuts: Loin chops, double lamb chops, T-bone chops, tenderloin.

Longer-cooking cuts: Loin of lamb.

Leg (Phases 1-4)
0 g Net Carbs

Versatile and fairly tender, leg of lamb is the most popular cut. Whole leg is the most economical (you may be able to talk the butcher into cutting off some chops from the sirloin), but the boneless ones cook quickly and are ideal for stuffing.

Quick-cooking cuts: Sirloin chops, leg steaks.

Longer-cooking cuts: Sirloin roast, whole sirloin, whole leg of lamb, half leg shank end, half leg sirloin end, butterflied leg (boneless), short leg (sirloin and hip bone removed).

Foreleg and Breast (Phases 1-4)
0 g Net Carbs

Cuts from the foreleg are called shank; they're tough, but braising makes them tender and brings out their wonderful flavor. The breast can include the spareribs and meat above the ribs; it too is delicious braised.

Quick-cooking cuts: Riblets.
Longer-cooking cuts: Shank, breast, spareribs.

➤ VEAL ◄

Like lamb, veal is a less popular choice than beef among Americans. Veal is high in protein and B vitamins; it's lower in fat and saturated fat than beef, mostly because it has very little marbling, or fat inside the muscle.

Veal, even from calves that are allowed to range freely, is quite tender; range-fed veal tends to be redder than stall-raised veal. Don't buy veal that is dark red or whitish pink. The former is on the old side, the latter will lack flavor. Fat should be white, ivory, or pale yellow, and the meat should be slightly moist but not mushy when you press it. And avoid veal preparations, like veal parmigiana and veal scallopini, which are floured and breaded and high in carbs.

Shoulder Cuts (Phases 1-4)
0 g Net Carbs

Veal shoulder, unlike shoulder from other animals, involves only the uppermost portion of the front of the animal (breast, and then shank, are the cuts lower on the front). Cuts from the shoulder are better browned, and then braised or pot-roasted.

Quick-cooking cuts: Veal blade steaks, veal arm steaks.

Longer-cooking cuts: Veal chuck neck off (boneless), veal chuck shoulder clod (boneless), veal blade roast, veal square, veal arm roast.

Rib Cuts (Phases 1-4)
0 g Net Carbs

Veal rib is from the back, just down from the shoulder. The rib can be cut into succulent, meaty chops or left whole for an impressive roast.

Quick-cooking cuts: Rib chops (boneless or bone-in), scallopini.

Longer-cooking cuts: Veal rib roast, rack.

Loin Cuts (Phases 1-4)
0 g Net Carbs

Veal loin is closer to the hip or leg, but unlike loin from other animals, veal loin can come from the belly as well as the back. Loin cuts are tender and flavorful; they are ideal sautéed, grilled, or roasted.

Quick-cooking cuts: Loin chops, top loin chops, veal kidney chops, scallopini.

Longer-cooking cuts: Veal loin roast.

Leg (Phases 1-4)
0 g Net Carbs

Veal leg corresponds to the sirloin and round from beef; cuts from the leg can dry out if overcooked because they are so lean.

Quick-cooking cuts: Sirloin veal steaks, scallopini.

Longer-cooking cuts: Sirloin roast, rump roast, veal round roast, leg of veal top roast, veal shank.

Breast (Phases 1-4)
0 g Net Carbs

Veal breast contains a considerable amount of connective tissue and is best braised (stuff beforehand with vegetables and cheese, if you like) or cubed for stews.

OVERLOOKED CUTS

For most of us, "meat" is a steak, a chop, or a roast—and that's too bad. There are plenty of cuts that often cost less and have better flavor than more common cuts. The only drawback is that some may require a long period of cooking over low heat to become tender, but a leisurely weekend (or a slow-cooker) provides a tidy solution.

- Oxtails and shanks are two beef cuts that make marvelous stews and soups. The meat from both is quite tough, but when braised it becomes tender and develops a rich beefy flavor.
- Pork provides a variety of overlooked cuts. In addition to leg of pork and picnic ham (from the shoulder), keep an eye out for ham hocks, either smoked or not; they're delicious cooked with sauerkraut. Instead of using hambone or bacon in a vegetable or bean soup, pick up some neck bones to use instead.
- Breast of lamb and breast of veal are both wonderful when stuffed or stewed.
- Variety meats and organ meats are often higher in nutrients than regular meats. Liver and sweetbreads, for example, are among the few animal foods that supply vitamin C; liver is particularly rich in vitamin A. If you think "shoe leather" when you hear "liver," know that this meat can be tender and delicious when cooked properly—quick sautéing, for example, prevents toughening. But opt for calves' liver, not beef liver. Pesticides, antibiotics, and other chemicals can accumulate in an animal's liver over time.

Foreleg (Phases 1-4)
0 g Net Carbs
Usually called veal shanks, the foreleg is always braised or stewed; one well-known preparation is *osso buco*, which

is veal shanks braised with olive oil, white wine, stock, onions, tomatoes, garlic, anchovies, carrots, celery and lemon peel.

➤ VARIETY MEATS ◄

Sometimes called organ meats or offal, variety meats are rich in iron and trace minerals like copper, zinc, and phosphorus, and in B vitamins. Liver, the most common organ meat, is extremely high in vitamins A and C.

If you're a fan of liver, look for calves' liver rather than beef liver. Calves' liver is more tender and milder in flavor. Because the liver acts as a "clearinghouse" for pesticides, fertilizers, antibiotics, and other chemicals, calves' liver is likely to harbor less of these than the liver of an older animal.

Organ meats are perishable; look to be sure they are carefully packaged, with no holes or tears in the wrapper. Plan to cook them the day you purchase them.

Calves' Liver (Phases 1-4)
0 g Net Carbs

Beef Liver (Phases 1-4)
0 g Net Carbs

Tongue (Phases 1-4)
0 g Net Carbs

Sweetbreads (Phases 1-4)
0 g Net Carbs

Pigs' Feet (Phases 1-4)
0 g Net Carbs

Tripe (Phases 1-4)
2 g Net Carbs

➤ GAME ◄

Not all supermarkets stock game, and it may be available seasonally in those that do. If you don't see it in your favorite store, ask the butcher if it can be ordered. Game is richly flavored and exceptionally lean.

Venison (Phases 1-4)
0 g Net Carbs
Leaner than beef, venison is an excellent alternative for red-meat lovers; it supplies generous amounts of B vitamins, iron, riboflavin, niacin, and zinc. Ranch-raised venison is less gamy than wild venison.

Buffalo (Phases 1-4)
0 g Net Carbs

Beefalo (Phases 1-4)
0 g Net Carbs
Look for steaks and roasts of these animals (beefalo is a cross between domestic cattle and bison); you may find ground buffalo, too. These meats are very lean and are best broiled or roasted.

Goat (Phases 1-4)
0 g Net Carbs
Like lamb, goat is milder in flavor and more tender when it is from younger animals; try goat in any recipe calling for lamb.

Rabbit (Phases 1-4)
0 g Net Carbs
Rabbit is higher in fat than most game, but it is still lower in fat and cholesterol than beef or dark chicken meat. Rabbit shares white-meat chicken's delicate flavor. Hare is comparable to dark meat and has a stronger flavor.

WHAT TO DO WITH LEFTOVERS

It's one thing when you've planned to have leftovers for a speedy supper later in the week, but one lonely pork chop is something else. When you have barely enough meat for a meal (or just enough for a serving), here are some suggestions so it won't go to waste:

BEEF

1. Cube leftover steak; heat with canned tomatoes and serve over 2 ounces Atkins Quick Quisine Pasta Cuts. (Phases 2-4; 7 g Net Carbs)
2. Cut into bite-size strips; arrange over ½ cup of mesclun and sprinkle with 2 tablespoons of crumbled blue cheese and your favorite controlled-carb dressing for a bistro-style salad. (Phases 1-4; 3 g Net Carbs)
3. Thinly slice; sear quickly just to heat through and serve alongside two eggs for a hearty breakfast. (Phases 1-4; 1 g Net Carbs)

PORK

1. Reheat slices of pork loin or leftover chops in liquid to keep them moist; broth, or a fruity white wine in later phases, is nice. (Phases 1-4; 1 g Net Carbs)
2. Cube leftover pork loin or fresh ham; add to broth made from water and a bouillon cube with ginger, garlic, shredded bok choy, bean sprouts, soy sauce, sesame oil, and pepper flakes for an Asian-inspired soup. (Phases 1-4; 2 g Net Carbs)
3. Sauté plenty of garlic in a little olive oil; remove from the heat and stir in 2 tablespoons lime juice, salt, cumin, and pepper. Pour over thin slices of roast pork for a Cuban-inspired entree. (Phases 1-4; 3 g Net Carbs)

LAMB

1. Cube or slice leftover lamb; toss with arugula, cherry or grape tomatoes, an ounce of feta cheese, and a zesty controlled-carb dressing *Tip: toss the salad with a teaspoon or so of beef broth before you dress it.* (Phases 1-4; 3 g Net Carbs)
2. Cut leftovers into large chunks. Sauté onion and garlic until golden, then add curry powder, cumin, cinnamon, and salt and cook until very aromatic. Add the lamb with some broth and ¼ cup of diced tomatoes and cook until the lamb is very tender. (Phases 1-4; 2 g Net Carbs)
3. Dice finely and sauté with low-carb vegetables; use to stuff a tomato or small zucchini. (Phases 1-4; 3 g Net Carbs)

VEAL

1. Sauté ½ cup mushrooms, then add thinly sliced veal. Add broth and vinegar and cook until the veal is heated through and the liquid is almost evaporated. (Phases 1-4; 2 g Net Carbs)
2. Cut into very small chunks; add to a ¼ cup tomato sauce and serve over 2 ounces of Atkins Quick Quisine Pasta Cuts. (Phases 2-4; 9 g Net Carbs)
3. Cut into thin strips, then sauté with 4 steamed asparagus spears. Serve sprinkled with lemon zest. (Phases 1-4; 2 g Net Carbs)

The Poultry Section

Like fish, shellfish, and meat, great-tasting, versatile, fresh poultry is one of the basic meal builders when you're doing Atkins. Fowl is high in B vitamins, iron, protein, and trace minerals like zinc and selenium, and it's completely free of carbohydrates.

Challenge yourself to look beyond chicken. Turkey, duck, and game hens are readily available whole or, in the case of duck and turkey, cut up.

If you buy a whole bird to roast, keep in mind that there's considerable waste: A 4- to 5-pound chicken will yield a little over a pound of cooked meat—enough for four, with a little left over. Larger birds tend to have more meat on them in relation to the bone. Boneless cuts are more expensive, but there's virtually no waste. Don't automatically reach for boneless breasts or thighs, though: Cuts cooked on the bone are often more flavorful.

Be especially wary of preseasoned poultry and heat-and-serve entrees. These can harbor hidden sugars and fillers.

➤ CHICKEN ◄

Chicken is an incredibly versatile source of protein, whether your meal is a formal Sunday dinner or a picnic buffet. Its relatively bland flavor marries well with a variety of seasonings and sauces—chicken can be used in place of pork in virtually all recipes, and in lieu of beef or fish in many.

Whole chickens are categorized by weight. Chicken parts are available by part or as a cut-up chicken—that is, two breasts, two thighs, two drumsticks, two wings, and the back. Here are some of the items you might find:

Whole Broiler-Fryers (Phases 1-4)
0 g Net Carbs
Weighing up to 3½ pounds, broiler-fryers are young, fairly lean, somewhat bland birds. Although they are often cut up for broiling or frying, they can be left whole and roasted.

Whole Roasters (Phases 1-4)
0 g Net Carbs
Roasters can weigh 5 or more pounds; they're higher in fat than broiler-fryers and have a richer flavor.

Capon (Phases 1-4)
0 g Net Carbs
These large—often weighing 10 pounds or so—birds are wonderfully flavorful and particularly suited to roasting. They have large breasts and are a terrific alternative to small turkeys, which often have little meat.

Breast (Phases 1-4)
0 g Net Carbs
Skinless, boneless breasts are ubiquitous, whether you buy them as thin-sliced cutlets (these cook ultra-fast), fingers (narrow strips of chicken, sometimes called chicken tenders), or boned and skinned breasts. You'll also find bone-in breasts, which take somewhat longer to cook but are much richer in flavor.

Thighs (Phases 1-4)
0 g Net Carbs
Dark meat is higher in fat than white meat chicken; therefore, it has a meatier flavor and juicier texture. Look for con-

venient boneless, skinless thighs and use them instead of chicken breasts in your favorite recipe.

Drumsticks (Phases 1-4)
0 g Net Carbs

Wings (Phases 1-4)
0 g Net Carbs
   These cuts have comparatively little meat on them, and if they're not cooked carefully can dry out rapidly. Try brushing wings with a controlled-carb spicy marinade for Buffalo wings and serve with homemade blue cheese dipping sauce (see *www.atkins.com* for recipes).

Rock Cornish Hens (Phases 1-4)
0 g Net Carbs
   These miniature chickens generally weigh ¾–1 pound each, with one hen enough for one portion. They're often roasted or split and broiled or grilled.

➤ TURKEY ◄

   There's no reason to limit turkey to the holidays—many supermarkets stock whole turkeys year-round. Even if you don't want a 16-pound bird, you can find whole breasts to roast, as well as thighs, drumsticks, cutlets and wings.
   Smaller turkeys can have little meat compared to the amount of bone they contain; if your Thanksgiving feast will be for a few, consider a capon or turkey breast instead of a smaller bird—you'll end up with a lot more meat.

Whole Turkey (Phases 1-4)
0 g Net Carbs
   Pass on the pre-basted turkeys—they're injected with a salty, fatty substance that keeps them moist while roasting (and it may contain sugar). You'll get better flavor and bet-

SAFE HANDLING:
MEAT, POULTRY, AND SEAFOOD

Animal products, like meat, poultry, and seafood, require special care during preparation and cooking. To prevent foodborne illnesses from bacteria found in these foods, follow these guidelines:

- Wash hands, cutting boards, dishes and utensils with hot soapy water before and after contact with raw meats.
- Use one cutting board for raw meats and one for fresh fruits and veggies.
- Keep raw meats away from other foods in your grocery cart, refrigerator and during preparation.
- Place cooked meats on a clean plate; do not use the same plate that held the food in its raw state. Do not reapply a marinade used on raw meats to the cooked item, unless the marinade has been boiled beforehand.
- Use a meat thermometer. Cook these raw meats to the following safe internal temperatures:
  Ground meat: 160° F
  Pork: 160° F (for medium); 170° F (well done)
  Poultry, whole: 180° F
  Poultry, breasts: 170° F
  Fish: Cook until opaque and flaky

ter nutrition by choosing an unadorned bird and basting it yourself.

Breast (Phases 1-4)
0 g Net Carbs
Whole, bone-in turkey breasts roast fairly rapidly so they're an ideal alternative to roast chicken. Look for turkey breast cutlets—boned, skinned, and sliced very thinly—to use in place of chicken breast.

Wings (Phases 1-4)
0 g Net Carbs

Drumsticks (Phases 1-4)
0 g Net Carbs

Somewhat meatier than chicken wings, turkey wings are about the size of a chicken drumstick. Wings and drumsticks are wonderful to use for soups and stews.

Ground (Phases 1-4)
0 g Net Carbs

Far more common than ground chicken, ground turkey is an alternative to beef. Problem is, because it has less fat, it's also less flavorful and trickier to cook. Avoid packages marked "skinless ground turkey breast"—the dark meat has more flavor, and the skin adds moisture and fat.

➤ DUCK ◄

When purchasing duck, look for a broad, somewhat plump breast. Duck is entirely dark meat and is high in niacin, iron, selenium, and protein. This versatile bird is delicious roasted, braised and broiled.

Whole Duck (Phases 1-4)
0 g Net Carbs

Duck doesn't contain much meat compared to bone—a 3- to 4-pound duck will feed two or three people. Whole duck is most often roasted, and it needs to be watched carefully as grease can accumulate in the roasting pan and may need to be spooned off lest it catch fire.

Breast (Phases 1-4)
0 g Net Carbs

Duck's rich flavor is closer to beef and dark-meat chicken than to chicken breast. Try using duck breast in place of steak in a recipe.

➤ GAME BIRDS ◄

Goose (Phases 1-4)
0 g Net Carbs
Very rich and quite fatty, goose supplies generous amounts of B vitamins, selenium, zinc, and iron. Like duck, it is entirely dark meat. It's most often available around the holidays, almost always as a whole bird.

Pheasant (Phases 1-4)
0 g Net Carbs
Among the leanest game birds, pheasant is an excellent source of protein and iron. Purchase one bird to serve two people, and cook it carefully to prevent it from drying out.

Ostrich (Phases 1-4)
0 g Net Carbs
Ostrich is sold in steaks and is comparable in flavor, texture, and color to lean beef or duck breast. Another very lean bird, it has about one-fifth the fat of dark chicken meat.

➤ SAUSAGE, LUNCH MEATS, AND CURED POULTRY ◄

Often marked as a lean alternative to beef and pork products, poultry sausages and cured meats frequently require more seasonings and additives to make them palatable. They should be treated with the same caveats that their meat-based counterparts are: Limit consumption of those cured with nitrates (often identifiable by their reddish coloring), and for the freshest products and best flavor, purchase meats from the deli counter (see page 66) rather than the lunch meat section.

KOSHER POULTRY: IS IT BETTER?

Even if you don't keep a kosher kitchen, you may wish to purchase kosher poultry. Kosher turkeys and chickens aren't more nutritious than non-kosher ones—in fact, they may be higher in sodium—but they have several advantages that make them worth their premium price.

Kosher birds are fed a special diet and are not given hormones. They are allowed to roam freely in a special indoor area that protects them from eating non-kosher items (but they are not considered free-range, because they are not outdoors). Processing a kosher bird takes about three times as long as processing a non-kosher bird, and many of the steps are performed by hand. The birds are salted and soaked, which enhances their flavor. In addition to USDA inspections, kosher birds must also pass inspection by rabbis.

Italian Sausage Turkey (Phases 1-4)
2.6 g Net Carbs per 2 ounces

Smoked Turkey Wings, Drumsticks, Tails (Phases 1-4)
1 g Net Carbs per 3 ounces

Turkey Pepperoni (Phases 1-4)
0 g Net Carbs per ounce (30 slices)

Turkey and Chicken Hot Dogs (Phases 1-4)
0-2 g Net Carbs per hot dog

Turkey Pastrami (Phases 1-4)
1 g Net Carbs per 2 ounces

Turkey Ham (Phases 1-4)
1 g Net Carbs per 2 ounces

Turkey Bacon (Phases 1-4)
1 g Net Carbs per 2 ounces

➤ PRESEASONED AND HEAT-AND-SERVE POULTRY ◀

Hate to cook? Looking for a few time-savers for crazy weeknights? Heat-and-serve poultry entrees may seem tempting, but you must choose carefully to avoid unnecessary carbs.

The product name is your first clue: Sweet and sour, barbecue, and teriyaki are tip-offs to added sugars; gravy signals added flour or starch. Anything breaded, wrapped in a tortilla, or with a crust is almost sure to be a Worst Bite. But that's not all you need to know to be sure unacceptable ingredients are not lurking in a dish—always ask someone in the poultry department for an ingredients list.

Chicken Alfredo (Phases 1-4)
3 g Net Carbs per 5 ounces

Homestyle with Gravy (Phases 2-4)
4 g Net Carbs per 5 ounces

Buffalo Wings (Phases 1-4)
1 g Net Carbs per 4 wings

Garlic Chicken (Phases 2-4)
7 g Net Carbs per cup

"Short Cut" Chicken Strips (Phases 1-4)
- **Original**   *2 g Net Carbs per ½ cup*
- **Southwestern**   *2 g Net Carbs per ½ cup*
- **Lemon-Pepper**   *2 g Net Carbs per ½ cup*
- **Italian**   *3 g Net Carbs per ½ cup*
- **Honey-Roasted**   *3 g Net Carbs per ½ cup*

Whole-Roasted Chicken (Phases 1-4)
1 g Net Carbs per 3 ounces

Italian-Style Chicken Meatballs (Phase 2-4)
4 g Net Carbs per 6 meatballs

SPOTLIGHT ON ORGANIC POULTRY

Organic foods, including organically raised chickens, are produced without antibiotics, artificial fertilizers and pesticides and other chemical additives, so eating them reduces your exposure to toxic substances that could harm your health. But did you know that organic foods are often more flavorful than their conventionally produced counterparts? Because they are typically locally grown, they are also often fresher and higher in nutrition.

Supporting organic farming goes beyond health and taste, however. By buying these products, you are helping to reduce the overall use of chemical fertilizers and pesticides, which in turn protects the environment. By buying organically produced poultry, eggs, milk and meat, you help reduce the agricultural use of antibiotics and hormones. Organic farming doesn't create the toxic runoff that pollutes water and disrupts ecosystems, and it helps preserve and improve farm soil.

WORST BITES: There may not be a Poultry Hall of Shame, but these foods are definitely the foulest of the fowl. Push your cart right past them.

- **Barbecued shredded chicken**   *11 g Net Carbs per ¼ cup*
- **Chicken nuggets**   *12 g Net Carbs per 4-5 nuggets*
- **Chicken cheese nuggets**   *13 g Net Carbs per 5 nuggets*
- **Barbecue turkey**   *16 g Net Carbs per 5 ounces*
- **Sweet and sour chicken**   *20 g Net Carbs per cup*
- **Chicken pies**   *29 g Net Carbs per pie*
- **Barbecue rotisserie chicken**   *34 g Net Carbs per 5 ounces*
- **Burritos**   *34 g Net Carbs per burrito*
- **Taquitos**   *37 g Net Carbs per 3 taquitos*

The Dairy Case

From nutrient-rich eggs to refrigerated cookie dough, the dairy case contains some of the best and worst choices in the supermarket—and to make your selection even trickier, some of the worst choices have a reputation for being nutritious: Regular fruit-flavored yogurt, for example, is full of sugar.

There are some sections of the refrigerated foods aisle that you can push your cart straight past—refrigerated biscuits and cookies and nonfat half-and-half are chock-full of sugars and hydrogenated oils. Whipped cream in cans and prepared puddings are unacceptably high in carbohydrates and may contain other unacceptable ingredients, like added sugars and hydrogenated oils.

➤ CHEESE ◄

Nutrients in cheese vary widely. Harder cheeses tend to be higher in protein and calcium, and lower in carbohydrates, than fresh and softer cheeses. In fact, most fresh cheeses such as cottage cheese, ricotta and farmer cheese, are not allowed on Induction; processed cheeses can be high in Net Carbs as well and may contain unacceptable fillers.

Up to 4 ounces of soft, semi-soft, semi-hard, and hard cheeses are permitted each day. If you don't have a scale, it's easy to eyeball an ounce. All but the hardest cheeses are about the size of two dice, or about ¼ cup of grated or crumbled cheese. An ounce of Parmesan or pecorino Romano, however, measures a little under a tablespoon when grated.

Remember, too, that whole-fat cheeses are always a better choice. Lower-fat cheeses will actually have a higher carbohydrate content than full-fat cheese.

FRESH CHEESE

When it comes to cheese, "fresh" means that the cheese has not been aged or ripened. These cheeses are more like milk than harder ones. They are comparatively high in carbohydrate, and they are quite perishable, so it's important to look at sell-by dates.

Cottage Cheese (Phases 2-4)
* **Whole Milk** *2.8 g Net Carbs per ½ cup*
* **2% Fat** *4.1 g Net Carbs per ½ cup*

Whether your preference is large or small curd cottage cheese, skip those that are reduced-fat or flavored with pineapple or packaged with fruit toppings. If you like fruit mixed in with your cottage cheese (and your CCLL is high enough), add some berries or other low-glycemic fresh fruit instead of the excessively sweetened fruit.

Cream Cheese, whipped or stick, plain (Phases 1-4)
0.8 g Net Carbs per 2 tablespoons
* **Chive and Onion (Phases 2-4)**
  2 g Net Carbs per 2 tablespoons
* **Neufchatel (Phases 2-4)**
  2 g Net Carbs per 2 tablespoons
* **⚠ Strawberry** *5 g Net Carbs per 2 tablespoons*
  Contains added sugars.

Only plain, full-fat, brick-style cream cheese is allowed during Induction—cream cheese spreads, reduced-fat cream cheese, and fruit-flavored cream cheese are not. Flavored cream cheese tends to be high in additives, so check ingredients labels carefully. You might be better off adding chopped fresh chives to cream cheese than picking up a tub of the flavored stuff. Neufchatel is a reduced-fat form of cream cheese.

Goat (Phases 1-4)
0.3 g Net Carbs per ounce

Sometimes called chèvre, goat cheese can range in texture from spreadably smooth to quite crumbly.

Mascarpone (Phases 1-4)
0.6 g Net Carbs per ounce

This ultra-rich Italian cheese is similar to soft butter in consistency. Mix it with mustard or anchovies and serve it with vegetables for a terrific dip. In OWL, it is wonderful served with berries.

Mozzarella (Phases 1-4)
- **Whole Milk** *0.6 g Net Carbs per ounce*
- **Part Skim** *0.8 g Net Carbs per ounce*

If you're lucky enough to shop at a market with a large cheese section, you may find balls of fresh mozzarella; they're often packed in plastic bags. Drizzle a slice or two with olive oil and sprinkle with fresh basil for a treat.

Ricotta (Phases 2-4)
- **Whole Milk** *1.9 g Net Carbs per ½ cup*
- **Part Skim** *3.2 g Net Carbs per ½ cup*

Originally made from the whey that drained off during the making of provolone and mozzarella, ricotta has a slightly sweet flavor and a somewhat grainy texture.

SOFT AND SEMISOFT CHEESE

Blue (Phases 1-4)
0.7 g Net Carbs per ounce; 0.4 g per 2 tablespoons

Gorgonzola (Phases 1-4)
0 g Net Carbs per ounce

Roquefort (Phases 1-4)
0.6 g Net Carbs per ounce
Blue cheeses can be mild or quite pungent. If you'll be cooking with it, choose a strongly flavored one like Roquefort or Stilton. Milder blues like Gorgonzola are ideal for sprinkling onto salads.

Boursin (Phases 1-4)
1.0 g Net Carbs per 2 tablespoons
This soft, creamy cheese is often seasoned with herbs.

Brie (Phases 1-4)
0.1 g Net Carbs per ounce

Camembert (Phases 1-4)
0.1 g Net Carbs per ounce
Brie and Camembert are covered with an edible rind that can be bitter. Both are perfectly ripe when they "ooze"—if they're runny, they're too ripe.

Edam (Phases 1-4)
0.4 g Net Carbs per ounce

Gouda (Phases 1-4)
0.6 g Net Carbs per ounce
Hailing from Holland, these cheeses are covered with an inedible wax; they have a mellow, somewhat nutty flavor. Serve them as part of a dessert course.

Feta (Phases 1-4)
1.2 g Net Carbs per ounce
Feta cheese is cured in a brine, so it's actually pickled. Because it's cured it isn't considered fresh, but it is nutri-

tionally similar to fresh cheeses. Feta, however, is allowed in Induction.

Havarti (Phases 1-4)
0.8 g Net Carbs per ounce
This mild Danish cheese is often flavored with caraway or dill.

Limburger (Phases 1-4)
0.1 g Net Carbs per ounce
Something of an acquired taste (and smell!), Limburger is a pungent cheese that's best served with foods that are equally strong in flavor, such as onions or highly seasoned sausages.

Monterey Jack (Phases 1-4)
0.2 g Net Carbs per ounce
Occasionally referred to simply as Jack, this cheese can be aged as briefly as one week or up to 10 months. Jack cheese melts beautifully, so it's wonderful to cook with; aged Jack makes a fine alternative to grated cheddar in many recipes.

Muenster (Phases 1-4)
0.3 g Net Carbs per ounce
If your supermarket has an extensive cheese section, you may find imported Muenster. These European cheeses are much more robust in flavor than their American counterparts.

Provolone (Phases 1-4)
0.6 g Net Carbs per ounce
Young provolone is recognizable by its whitish color and mild flavor; aged provolone has a sharp, pungent bite and is creamier, almost yellow, in color. Aged provolone is a delicious alternative to cheddar or Parmesan.

HARD AND SEMIHARD CHEESE

Cheddar (Phases 1-4)
0.4 g Net Carbs per ounce

Colby (Phases 1-4)
0.7 g Net Carbs per ounce
Cheddar is the most popular cheese in the United States, and for good reason: It melts beautifully and is available from mild to extra sharp. Colby is a type of cheddar; its flavor is quite mild.

Fontina (Phases 1-4)
0.4 g Net Carbs per ounce
Originally from northern Italy, fontina is now made in several European countries as well as in the United States. Fontina melts well and works for almost any recipe. It's worth seeking out the Italian variety, though—it's more flavorful.

Manchego (Phases 1-4)
1 g Net Carbs per ounce
Spain's best-known cheese, manchego has a rich yet creamy texture. It's delicious as a snack and melts beautifully.

Parmesan (Phases 1-4)
0.9 g Net Carbs per ounce; 0.2 g per tablespoon

Romano (Phases 1-4)
1 g Net Carbs per ounce; 0.2 g per tablespoon
Parmesan and Romano are hard cheeses from Italy that are ideal for grating or shaving over stews and soups. Parmesan is made from cow's milk, but the most commonly available Romano is pecorino, a sharply flavored cheese similar to Parmesan that's made of sheep's milk.

Swiss (Phases 1-4)
1.0 g Net Carbs per ounce

Like cheddar and blue cheese, Swiss cheese is an extensive family that includes Emmental (sometimes called Emmentaler) and Gruyère; Jarlsberg is a Swiss-style cheese from Norway. Instantly recognizable by its large holes, Swiss cheese has a nutty flavor and melts beautifully.

PROCESSED CHEESE

Often labeled "cheese food," processed cheeses are higher in additives and carbohydrate than aged cheeses are. Read ingredients labels carefully.

American Singles (Phases 1-4)
0.3 g Net Carbs per slice (⅔ ounce)

Cold Pack Cheese Food (Phases 2-4)
2.4 g Net Carbs per 2 tablespoons

Laughing Cow (Phases 1-4)
1 g Net Carbs per wedge

String Cheese (Phases 1-4)
1 g Net Carbs per string

Kraft Velveeta Cheese (Phases 2-4)
3 g Net Carbs per ounce

⚠ Kraft Cheez Whiz
4 g Net Carbs per 2 tablespoons

Contains added sugars.

GRATED CHEESE

Supermarkets stock bags of grated or shredded cheese both singly—cheddar only, mozzarella only—or in blends for specific cuisines or dishes (Taco blend, Italian blend). Grated cheese spoils more rapidly than do blocks of cheese; if properly wrapped, a block of cheese may keep for several months, but once you've opened a bag of cheese, you have a week or so before it begins to moulder.

You're also at the mercy of what size and shape a manufacturer decides the cheese shavings should be—and many are perfect rectangles, so they don't melt prettily—and what they consider an optimal blend.

Most types (Phases 1-4)
1 g Net Carbs per ¼ cup

➤ DIPS AND SALSA ◄

Stocked near the sour cream, packaged dip is full of unpronounceable ingredients as well as sweeteners and partially hydrogenated vegetable oil, a form of trans fats, which means this is never an acceptable food in any phase of Atkins. Anyway, you'll get better flavor and fewer additives if you purchase sour cream and stir in your own seasonings.

Hummus, the Middle Eastern dip made of chickpeas and seasonings, is high in fiber and makes for fast snacks or light meals. Prepared tubs can be pricey; you can make it from scratch with chickpeas and tahini for pennies.

You may find salsas near tortillas and cheeses in the refrigerator case as well. Read the labels carefully. Some brands contain sugar (usually in the form of high-fructose corn syrup) and should be avoided. Green salsa, made from tomatillos, tends to be lower in carbs. Acceptable brands include Santa Barbara, Garden of Eatin' and Parker's Farm.

⚠ **French Onion Dip, most brands**
3 g Net Carbs per 2 tablespoons
  Contains trans fats.

⚠ **Green Onion Dip, most brands**
3 g Net Carbs per 2 tablespoons
  Contains trans fats.

⚠ **Horseradish Dip, most brands**
2 g Net Carbs per 2 tablespoons
  Contains trans fats.

Hummus (Phases 2-4)
2 g Net Carbs per 2 tablespoons

⚠ **Ranch Dip, most brands**
2 g Net Carbs per 2 tablespoons
  Contains trans fats.

Salsa (Phases 1-4)
2 g Net Carbs per 2 tablespoons
  May contain added sugars.

➤ BREADS, DOUGH, AND BAKERY PRODUCTS ◄

As you might expect, refrigerated cookie dough, biscuit dough, and sweet roll cylinders are Worst Bites—not only are they full of sugars and loaded with carbs (even those for corn bread), but they also contain trans fats in the form of partially hydrogenated oils. Skip the bags of pizza dough, too. It's made with bleached flour.

If your market doesn't stock controlled-carb tortillas, reach for the corn tortillas—they are an acceptable choice in the later phases of Atkins and lower in carbs than the flour ones.

Atkins Bakery Tortillas (Phases 2-4)
5 g Net Carbs per tortilla

La Tortilla Factory (Phases 1-4)
3 g Net Carbs per 6-inch tortilla

Tortillas, regular (Phases 3 & 4)
- **Corn** *10.7 g Net Carbs per 6-inch tortilla*
- **FYI** Flour *15 g Net Carbs per 6-inch tortilla*
  Contains white flour.
- **Whole-wheat** *18.1 g Net Carbs per 6-inch tortilla;
  27 g per 8-inch*

➤ BUTTER, MARGARINE, AND SPREADS ◄

Expect to see huge changes in this section of the supermarket in the next few years. Most margarines are very high in dangerous trans fats in the form of manufactured hydrogenated oils (the minute amounts of natural trans fats that occur in dairy products are not of concern). By law, manufacturers will have to add trans fats information to the Nutrition Facts labels by 2006, and it's likely that many will reformulate their products rather than risk losing consumers who are concerned about the health risks of these fats. There are margarines made without hydrogenated oils, which can be found in natural foods stores and some supermarkets. The front panel of the package will specify that it is "trans fat free."

Another problem with margarine is that its fat content can vary, and if you grab the wrong type, your cooking may suffer. Butter and stick margarines are 80 percent fat, and most recipes are formulated with the assumption that you'll be using one of these. Never choose a soft, tub-style margarine or spread, or one that's reduced-fat. Also, pass on margarine-butter blends, which contain hydrogenated oils. If you are a confirmed margarine lover, look into trans fat-free margarine-yogurt blends.

Natural, creamy and unmistakable in flavor, butter remains the spread of choice for people controlling their carbohydrates. Butter provides a mix of saturated and unsaturated fats, and its flavor is inimitable. Unsalted butter is often fresher than salted butter—salt is a preservative, so salted butter may stay on warehouse or refrigerator shelves longer.

Butter (Phases 1-4)
0 g Net Carbs per tablespoon
   Whether you choose whipped, salted, or unsalted butter, you'll get unparalleled flavor. Don't use whipped butter in most recipes, though—it has air mixed into it, so it has less fat by volume and will not give the same results.

 Margarine, regular
   Contains trans fats.
   • **⚠ Fat-Free Bottle** *0.8 g Net Carbs per tablespoon*
   Contains trans fats.
   • **⚠ Fat-Free Spread** *0.6 g Net Carbs per tablespoon*
   Contains trans fats.
   Margarine labeling can be tricky: You'll see labels trumpeting that it's "cholesterol-free!" but don't be duped. Margarine never had cholesterol—but it can contain artery-damaging hydrogenated oils, which your body cannot digest. Look instead for boxes touting a trans fat-free margarine. Those that contain hydrogenated oils are a Worst Bite. (If the box doesn't say, look for the words "hydrogenated" or "partially hydrogenated" in the ingredients list.)

Cholesterol-Lowering Margarines (Phases 1-4)
   • **Smart Balance Buttery Spread**
   0 g Net Carbs per tablespoon
   • **⚠ Benecol Spread** *0 g Net Carbs per tablespoon*
   Contains trans fats.

> 🔄 **WORST BITES:** The "alternative spreads" below ALL contain hydrogenated oils, so don't be fooled by their healthier sounding names or ingredients, like yogurt and olive oil. Use butter instead.
>
> • **Brummel & Brown** *0 g Net Carbs per tablespoon*
>   **Spread**
> • **Shed's Spread** *0 g Net Carbs per tablespoon*
>   **Country Crock**
> • **Olivio** *0 g Net Carbs per tablespoon*

➤ MILK, CREAM, AND MILK SUBSTITUTES ◄

Milk is high in carbs and is not acceptable during Induction. Keep an eye out for a new category of controlled-carb dairy drinks that taste like milk; Atkins-Approved Hood Carb Countdown Dairy Beverage, for example, is available in whole-fat and low-fat formulations, as well as chocolate-flavored. These are fine during Induction and can be used just as you would regular milk. If you decide to switch to milk during the later phases of Atkins, opt for whole milk over a lower-fat variety. The less fat dairy products contain, the higher they are in carbohydrate. The same principle holds true for creams: Whipping cream is lower in Net Carbs than is half-and-half. On Atkins, you should always opt for the higher-fat choices.

Avoid nondairy creamers (especially the flavored ones), fat-free half-and-half, and flavored milks. Full of sugar (usually in the form of high-fructose corn syrup) and hydrogenated oils, these unacceptable beverages qualify as Worst Bites. The exception is soy creamers. You may choose to use unsweetened soy-based creamers, such as White Wave Silk Creamer with 1 gram of Net Carbs per serving, for your coffee or tea (see page 125 for soymilk options).

Milk (Phases 3 & 4)
- **Whole** *11.4 g Net Carbs per cup*
- **Buttermilk** *13 g Net Carbs per cup*
- **Lowfat (1%)** *11.7 g Net Carbs per cup*
- **Nonfat, Skim** *11.9 g Net Carbs per cup*
- **Reduced Fat (2%)** *11.7 g Net Carbs per cup*
- **Lactaid, Skim** *13 g Net Carbs per cup*
- **Lactaid, Whole** *12 g Net Carbs per cup*
- **Calcium-Fortified** *12 g Net Carbs per cup*

CONTROLLED-CARB DAIRY BEVERAGES

Atkins-Approved Hood Carb Countdown Dairy Beverage, whole, 2%, chocolate (Phases 1-4)
3 g Net Carbs per cup

LeCarb Dairy Drink (Phases 2-4)
- **Whole** *4 g Net Carbs per cup*
- **2%** *4.5 g Net Carbs per cup*
- **Chocolate** *6 g Net Carbs per cup*

CREAM

Be sure to limit your intake of heavy cream to 3 ounces a day; cream can slow down weight loss, so if you aren't progressing as quickly as you'd like, you may wish to avoid it until you're out of Induction.

Up to an ounce (2 tablespoons) of sour cream per day is allowed during Induction, but only the full-fat variety. Light sour cream is made with half-and-half. Don't use it when cooking as it may curdle. Crème fraiche is an aged, thickened cream with a tangy-nutty flavor and the texture of sour cream; it's terrific for adding creaminess to soups and sauces since it doesn't curdle.

Half-and-Half (Phases 1-4)
0.5 g Net Carbs per tablespoon

Heavy Cream (Phases 1-4)
0.3 g Net Carbs per tablespoon

Heavy Cream, whipped (Phases 1-4)
0.3 g Net Carbs per 2 tablespoons

Light Cream (Phases 1-4)
0.4 g Net Carbs per tablespoon

Full-Fat Sour Cream (Phases 1-4)
1.2 g Net Carbs per 2 tablespoons

Light Sour Cream (Phases 2-4)
2 g Net Carbs per 2 tablespoons

Crème Fraiche (Phases 1-4)
1 g Net Carbs per ounce

SOYMILK

Often touted as a healthful alternative to cow's milk, some brands of soymilk can contain twice the grams of Net Carbs of cow's milk. First of all, soybeans contain carbohydrate, and even though you won't often see "sugar" or "high-fructose corn syrup" in the ingredients list, the overwhelming majority of soy beverages are sweetened with barley syrup, rice syrup, or cane juice.

Look for the word "unsweetened" on the label, or choose one with no more than 5 grams of Net Carbs per cup.

Moo (Not!), Low Sugar (Phases 1-4)
1 g Net Carbs per cup

⚠ **Plain or Vanilla, most brands**
10 g Net Carbs per cup
   Contains added sugars.

Unsweetened, most brands (Phases 1-4)
4-5 g Net Carbs per cup

⚠ White Wave Silk Nog
15 g Net Carbs per ½ cup
  Contains added sugars.

**White Wave Silk Organic Soymilk, unsweetened
(Phases 1-4)**
4 g Net Carbs per cup

White Wave Silk Soymilk Creamer (Phases 1-4)
1 g Net Carbs per tablespoon

➤ YOGURT AND SMOOTHIES ◀

High in calcium, protein, vitamins, and minerals, at its
best, yogurt is comparable to milk in carbohydrate. But flavored yogurts are downright treacherous: Some contain the
equivalent of 2 tablespoons of sugar per 8-ounce container—
it isn't unusual for fruit-flavored yogurts to weigh in with 40
grams of Net Carbs! Typical drinkable yogurts and yogurt
smoothies can have up to 60 grams of Net Carbs in a 10–11-
ounce bottle. Even sugar-free flavored yogurts can supply
close to 20 grams of Net Carbs.

Because fruit takes up space in a yogurt cup, you're getting less calcium if you buy fruit-flavored yogurts. An 8-
ounce tub of plain yogurt contains nothing but yogurt. An
8-ounce tub of fruit-flavored yogurt contains yogurt, sugar,
fruit, corn syrup, cornstarch, and a host of emulsifiers and
enhancers.

Look for the newest additions to the yogurt market—there
are now several brands of controlled-carb yogurts out there.
If you choose regular yogurt, in later phases, buy plain yogurt made with whole milk. Stir in berries and wheat germ
for a little crunch.

YOGURT

Atkins-Approved Hood Carb Countdown Reduced Sugar Low-Fat Yogurt, French Vanilla (Phases 1-4)
2 g Net Carbs per 6 ounces

Atkins-Approved Hood Carb Countdown Reduced Sugar Low-Fat Yogurt, Blueberry, Raspberry, Strawberry-Banana (Phases 1-4)
3 g Net Carbs per 6 ounces
   (Note: Product does not contain enough fruit to impact blood sugar.)

Blue Bunny Carb Freedom Yogurt, Peach, Raspberry, Strawberry, Vanilla Crème (Phases 2-4)
5 g Net Carbs per 6 ounces

LeCarb YoCarb, Plain (Phases 1-4)
3 g Net Carbs per 4 ounces

LeCarb YoCarb, Lemon, Peach Mango, Strawberry-Banana, Key Lime, Blueberry (Phases 2-4)
4 g Net Carbs per 4 ounces

Dannon Light 'n Fit Carb Control, Peaches 'n Cream, Raspberries 'n Cream, Strawberries 'n Cream, Vanilla Cream (Phases 1-4)
3 g Net Carbs per 4 ounces

Plain, Whole Milk, most brands (Phases 3 & 4)
11 g Net Carbs per 8 ounces

Plain, Low-Fat, most brands (Phases 3 & 4)
15 g Net Carbs per 8 ounces

SMOOTHIES

Look for controlled-carb ready-to-drink smoothies or make your own by blending controlled-carb yogurt, frozen berries and/or ice (thin as needed with water).

⚠ **Dannon Light 'n Fit Smoothies, Mixed Berry, Peach Passion Fruit, Raspberry, Strawberry, Strawberry-Banana, Tropical**
14-15 g Net Carbs per 7-fluid ounce container
Contains added sugars.

ORGANIC ACIDS

Organic acids are found in most fermented foods and in tangy or sour foods such as orange juice or sauerkraut, respectively. Fermented meat, such as pepperoni and luncheon meats, also contain organic acids, as does most fruit, sour cream, yogurt, buttermilk and cheesecake. On food labels, organic acids are considered part of the total carbohydrates but are not broken out. They do not have a significant impact on blood sugar and therefore do not count as Net Carbs.

➤ EGGS ◄

Eggs are a terrific source of protein, vitamins, and minerals. Most of the carbohydrate, cholesterol, fat, and fat-soluble vitamins are in the yolk; the white contains the protein, water, and most of the minerals. "Enhanced" eggs supply omega-3 fatty acids and vitamin E.

If a recipe, such as Caesar salad dressing, calls for raw eggs and you're concerned about foodborne illness, you may choose to use egg substitutes, which are made primarily of egg whites.

Eggs (Phases 1-4)
0.6 g Net Carbs per large egg

Egg Whites (Phases 1-4)
0.4 g Net Carbs per large egg white

Egg Substitutes (Phases 1-4)
0.5-1 g Net Carbs per ½ cup

➤ JUICES ◄

Juice contains all the carbohydrate of a fruit (sometimes more, if sugar or corn syrup has been added) and none of the fiber. Eat the whole fruit instead of pouring a glass of juice and you'll get the benefit of the fiber, which slows down the impact of the sugar on your bloodstream.

If you must have juice, tomato and grapefruit are your best bets. Most other fruit juices—even unsweetened ones—weigh in with 30 grams of Net Carbs or more per 4-ounce serving and, frankly, it's probably not worth spending carbs on. To bring juice more in line, use just a splash in your water or dilute it with seltzer for a refreshingly light beverage.

Apple, unsweetened (Phases 3 & 4)
29 g Net Carbs per cup

Cranberry, unsweetened (Phases 3 & 4)
31 g Net Carbs per cup

Grapefruit, white or pink (Phases 3 & 4)
23 g Net Carbs per cup

Orange (Phases 3 & 4)
26 g Net Carbs per cup

Orange Blend (Phases 3 & 4)
30 g Net Carbs per cup

➤ REFRIGERATED SNACKS ◄

High in sugars and modified starches, packaged puddings are a Worst Bite; low-fat and fat-free varieties abound, but sugar-free ones are few and far between.

WORST BITES: Turn to the dairy case for milk, but don't get your cookies—or biscuits, breadsticks, or cinnamon rolls—here. Refrigerated doughs range from 11–30 grams of Net Carbs per biscuit, and they're loaded with hydrogenated oils, too.

Skip the fat-free flavored creamers and half-and-half. Both are loaded with thickeners and fats; flavored creamer has more than 10 times the Net Carbs of regular half-and-half.

Soymilk can be a nutritious, controlled-carb alternative to cow's milk, but stay with the unsweetened varieties. Chocolate soymilk has almost six times the Net Carbs of unsweetened soymilk.

Most regular smoothies and drinkable yogurts win the "Hall of Shame" Worst Bite Award. With as many as 60 grams of Net Carbs in an 11-ounce bottle, these are a far cry from the healthful beverages they're touted to be. Whip up smoothies at home with fresh fruit, tofu, and sucralose, or choose a controlled-carb version instead.

➤ THE INTERIOR ◄

Prepared foods from canned soup to cold cereal make up the lion's share of the interior aisles of most supermarkets. Here's the skinny on what's okay to add to your cart and what should stay on the shelves.

The Cookies and Crackers Aisle

Added sugar and bleached white flour are no strangers to the cookies and crackers aisle, so both areas can be particularly challenging when you're searching for controlled-carb products. Plus, virtually all major brands use dangerous hydrogenated oils, so even sugar-free cookies can contain this form of heart-damaging trans fats, which are absolute no-nos on Atkins; in fact, they should be avoided at all costs no matter what your dietary regimen.

During Induction, don't waste your time in this aisle. In Ongoing Weight Loss, the selection will increase slightly, but only in the latter phases of Atkins will you find more options here. Keep in mind, your choices will still be limited even when your Net Carb threshold increases, since hydrogenated oils and added sugar must always be avoided. To make the best picks here, go with items that offer a lot of flavor and a great texture—cookies with these qualities will be more likely to satisfy you in fewer bites.

Your best bets: For crackers, look for flatbreads. Many are made with rye, and some are exceptionally high in fiber. Others are fat free—careful here, since they can contain sugar; however, you won't have to worry about hydrogenated oils. For cookies, look for meringues, wafers, and treats made from nutritious whole grains such as oats and barley. If your market has a natural foods section, look there for trans fat-free cookies and crackers or visit your neighborhood natural foods store for other options (see pages 316 and 323).

➤ COOKIES AND BAKED GOODS ◄

Atkins Endulge Chewy Chocolate Chip Cookie Bites (Phases 2-4)
5 g Net Carbs per serving

Atkins Endulge Fudge Nut Brownies (Phases 2-4)
3 g Net Carbs per brownie

BP Gourmet Sugar-Free Chocolate Chip (Phases 3 & 4)
5 g Net Carbs per 4 cookies

BP Gourmet Vanilla Meringues (Phases 3 & 4)
7 g Net Carbs per 4 cookies

Heavenly Desserts Original Meringue, most flavors (Phases 1-4)
0 g Net Carbs per cookie

⚠ **Archway Sugar-Free Oatmeal**
8 g Net Carbs per cookie
  Contains trans fats.

⚠ **Archway Sugar-Free Peanut Butter**
7 g Net Carbs per cookie
  Contains trans fats.

⚠ **Archway Sugar-Free Rocky Road**
6 g Net Carbs per cookie
  Contains trans fats.

FYI Aunt Gussie's Sugar-Free Wheat Cookies, Chocolate Chip (Phases 3 & 4)
3 g Net Carbs per cookie
   Contains wheat flour.

FYI Aunt Gussie's Sugar-Free Choc-Chip Wheat Biscotti, Almond, Hazelnut, Raisin Almond (Phases 3 & 4)
7 Net Carbs per cookie
   Contains wheat flour.

FYI Aunt Gussie's Sugar-Free Oatmeal, Whole-Wheat (Phases 3 & 4)
8 g Net Carbs per cookie
   Contains wheat flour.

FYI Aunt Gussie's Sugar-Free Pecan Meltaways (Phases 3 & 4)
5 g Net Carbs per cookie
   Contains wheat flour.

⚠ Fifty-50 Chocolate Chip
9 g Net Carbs per 4 cookies
   Contains trans fats.

⚠ Fifty-50 Oatmeal
13 g Net Carbs per 4 cookies
   Contains trans fats.

⚠ Fifty-50 Chocolate Crème Sugar-Free Wafers
12 g Net Carbs per 6 wafers
   Contains trans fats.

⚠ Health Valley Oatmeal Cookies, Chocolate Chip, Raisin, Peanut Crunch
13 g Net Carbs per cookie
   Contains added sugars.

FYI Joseph's Sugar-Free Cookies, most flavors
(Phases 3 & 4)
13-15 g Net Carbs per 4 cookies
 Contains wheat flour.

⚠ Miss Meringue, Vanilla, Cappuccino, Natural
Lemon, Chocolate Chip, Mint Chocolate Chip
20 g Net Carbs per 4 cookies
 Contains added sugars.

⚠ Murray Sugar-Free Double Fudge Chewy
12 g Net Carbs per 3 cookies
 Contains trans fats.

⚠ Murray Sugar-Free Fudge Dipped Shortbread,
Vanilla Wafers
11 g Net Carbs per 3 cookies
 Contains trans fats and aspartame.

⚠ Murray Sugar-Free Lemon Cremes Sandwich,
Chocolate Chip
13 g Net Carbs per 3 cookies
 Contains trans fats.

⚠ Murray Sugar-Free Oatmeal
15 g Net Carbs per 3 cookies
 Contains trans fats.

⚠ Nabisco Arrowroot Biscuit
4 g Net Carbs per cookie
 Contains added sugars and trans fats.

⚠ Nabisco Zwieback Toast
6 g Net Carbs per cookie
 Contains added sugars and trans fats.

⚠ **SnackWell's Sugar-Free Oatmeal**
9 g Net Carbs per cookie
  Contains added sugars.

⚠ **SnackWell's Shortbread**
17 g Net Carbs per 3 cookies
  Contains trans fats and added sugars.

⚠ **Sorbee Zero Sugar Sandwich Cookies, Chocolate, Duplex**
8 g Net Carbs per 2 cookies
  Contains trans fats.

FYI **Sweet'N Low Wafers, Chocolate, Peanut Butter (Phases 3 & 4)**
21 g Net Carbs per 3 wafers
  Contains wheat flour.

SPOTLIGHT ON SUGAR ALCOHOLS

Also known as polyols, sugar alcohols are sugar molecules with hydroxy (or alcohol) groups attached. Sugar alcohols, such as maltitol, isomalt, sorbitol and lactitol, have many of the characteristics of carbohydrates. For instance, they serve to bulk up and sweeten foods. However, they provide fewer calories and do not impact blood glucose as does sugar. When determining the Net Carb count for foods containing sugar alcohols, subtract the grams of fiber as well as the grams of sugar alcohols from the grams of total carbohydrates.

Like sugar alcohols, glycerine does not impact blood sugar and therefore is not included in the Net Carb count.

➤ CRACKERS AND BREADSTICKS ◄

Andre's Carbo Save, all flavors (Phases 2-4)
4 g Net Carbs per 3 crackers

Blue Diamond Nut Thins (Phases 3 & 4)
20 g Net Carbs per 16 crackers

Devonsheer Melba Toast (Phases 3 & 4)
10 g Net Carbs per 3 pieces

Finn Crisp Rye Crispbread (Phases 3 & 4)
8 g Net Carbs per 3 slices

⚠ **Heavenly Desserts Gourmet Cracker, Sesame & Whole Wheat**
2.5 g Net Carbs per cracker
  Contains trans fats.

Kavli Thin Crispbread (Phases 3 & 4)
11 g Net Carbs per 3 pieces

Kavli Five-Grain Crispbread (Phases 2-4)
7 g Net Carbs per piece

⚠ **Nabisco Sociables**
9 g Net Carbs per 5 crackers
  Contains trans fats.

⚠ **Nabisco Royal Lunch Milk Crackers**
8 g Net Carbs per cracker
  Contains added sugars and trans fats.

⚠ **Nabisco Wheat Thins**
20 g Net Carbs per 16 crackers
  Contains added sugars and trans fats.

FYI **Old London Melba Toast (Phases 3 & 4)**
10 g Net Carbs per 3 pieces
  Contains flour.

Ryvita Original Wheat Crackerbread (Phases 3 & 4)
10 g Net Carbs per 3 slices

Ryvita Crispbread, Original, Dark Rye, Sesame, Multigrain, Flavorful Fiber (Phases 3 & 4)
12 g Net Carbs per 2 slices

Ryvita Light Rye Crispbread (Phases 3 & 4)
12 g Net Carbs per 2 slices

Ryvita Toasted Sesame Crispbread (Phases 3 & 4)
11 g Net Carbs per 2 slices

⚠ **Stella D'oro Breadsticks, Original**
7 g Net Carbs per breadstick
  Contains added sugars.

⚠ **Stella D'oro Breadsticks, Sesame, Roasted Garlic**
6 g Net Carbs per breadstick
  Contains added sugars.

Wasa Fiber Light Rye (Phases 3 & 4)
5 g Net Carbs per slice

Wasa Soya Crispbread (Phases 3 & 4)
6 g Net Carbs per slice

Wasa Fiber Rye Crispbread (Phases 2-4)
5 g Net Carbs per slice

Wasa Hearty Rye Crispbread (Phases 3 & 4)
10 g Net Carbs per slice

FABULOUS FLATBREADS

Craving a crunch? These slender crackers can satisfy your
yen. Most have a high-fiber content that keeps the grams of
Net Carbs at less than 10 per serving—sometimes even as
low as 4. With a little cream cheese and smoked salmon,
you've got yourself a great snack. But still, some brands are
higher in carbs and contain unacceptable ingredients, so
don't assume it's okay just because it's called flatbread: Read
the Nutrition Facts labels and avoid bleached white flour.

The Breakfast Foods Aisle

Mom was right, and now research backs her up: Breakfast is the most important meal of the day. Not only will a satisfying breakfast that's high in protein and low in carbs give you loads of energy to tide you over until lunchtime and help you think more clearly, but eating breakfast also makes it easier to lose weight and helps curb snacking.

The question, of course, is what constitutes a "good" controlled-carb breakfast. When it comes to cold cereal, most are loaded with sugar even those that are marketed as "healthy" and don't taste sweet usually contain at least some added sugar (even many bran cereals!), making them unacceptable on any phase of Atkins. Look for natural cereals that do not contain added sugars of any kind (including honey and corn syrup) and that are high in fiber, which helps you to stay fuller longer. Sugar-laden frosted toaster pastries are obviously out of the question, as are most regular and low-fat muffins, frozen waffles and pancakes. Ditto for bagels.

Think your only options are eggs? Think again. These days, there is an increasing number of terrific-tasting controlled-carb options that can help you wake up right.

➤ CEREAL ◄

COLD CEREAL

Sugars and hydrogenated oils packed into one convenient box—almost all of the foods in this aisle qualify as Worst Bites. Your best bets: Multigrain cereals, which typically have the highest amount of fiber. Seek out varieties with "multigrain" in the name, then check to see that they have at least 5 grams of fiber per serving—but also zoom in on the ingredients lists, since sugar in all its forms (cane juice, concentrated fruit juice, honey) may still be lurking inside.

Don't get fooled by serving sizes, either: Yes, they're all over the map, but they almost need to be. Bran cereals, for example, are very dense—you probably wouldn't want to sit down to a 1-cup serving. Puffed wheat, on the other hand, is full of air; ⅓ cup of it might be enough to bring its Net Carbs in line, but it won't be enough to provide you with the nutrients you need to start your day. When it comes to granola cereals, visit the natural foods store to find sugar-free or controlled-carb versions. (See other cold cereal options on page 310.)

Atkins Morning Start Cereal, Crunchy Almond Crisp (Phases 2-4)
3 g Net Carbs per ⅔ cup

Atkins Morning Start Cereal, Blueberry Bounty (Phases 2-4)
4 g Net Carbs per ⅔ cup

Atkins Morning Start Cereal, Banana Nut Harvest (Phases 2-4)
5 g Net Carbs per ⅔ cup

Alpen No Added Sugar or Salt (Phases 3 & 4)
26 g Net Carbs per ⅔ cup

⚠ **General Mills Cheerios**
19 g Net Carbs per cup
   Contains added sugars.

ℹ️ **General Mills Fiber One (Phases 2-4)**
10 g Net Carbs per ½ cup
   Contains aspartame.

⚠ **General Mills Kix**
24 g Net Carbs per 1⅓ cups
   Contains added sugars.

⚠ **General Mills Total, Whole Grain**
21 g Net Carbs per ¾ cup
   Contains added sugars.

⚠ **General Mills Wheaties**
21 g Net Carbs per cup
   Contains added sugars and trans fats.

⚠ **Health Valley Organic Fiber 7 Multigrain Flakes**
21 g Net Carbs per ¾ cup
   Contains added sugars.

⚠ **Health Valley Organic Oat Bran Flakes**
21 g Net Carbs per ¾ cup
   Contains added sugars.

⚠ **Health Valley Original Soy O's**
27 g Net Carbs per cup
   Contains added sugars.

⚠ **Kashi Go Lean**
18 g Net Carbs per ¾ cup
   Contains added sugars.

⚠️ Kashi Heart to Heart
20 g Net Carbs per ¾ cup
  Contains added sugars.

Kashi Puffed (Phases 3 & 4)
14 g Net Carbs per cup

⚠️ Kellogg's All-Bran, Original
11 g Net Carbs per ⅓ cup
  Contains added sugars.

⚠️ Kellogg's All-Bran, Extra Fiber
7 g Net Carbs per ½ cup
  Contains added sugars.

⚠️ Kellogg's Complete Oat Bran Flakes
19 g Net Carbs per ¾ cup
  Contains added sugars.

⚠️ Kellogg's Complete Wheat Bran Flakes
18 g Net Carbs per ¾ cup
  Contains added sugars.

⚠️ Kellogg's Corn Flakes
23 g Net Carbs per cup
  Contains added sugars.

⚠️ Kellogg's Corn Pops
28 g Net Carbs per cup
  Contains added sugars.

⚠️ Kellogg's Product 19
24 g Net Carbs per cup
  Contains added sugars.

⚠ **Kellogg's Rice Krispies**
29 g Net Carbs per 1¼ cups
  Contains added sugars.

⚠ **Kellogg's Special K**
22 g Net Carbs per cup
  Contains added sugars.

⚠ **Nutritious Living Hi-Lo**
5 g Net Carbs per ½ cup
  Contains added sugars.

Organic Weetabix (Phases 3 & 4)
24 g Net Carbs per 2 biscuits

⚠ **Post Bran Flakes**
19 g Net Carbs per ¾ cup
  Contains added sugars.

FYI **Post Grape-Nuts (Phases 3 & 4)**
41 g Net Carbs per ½ cup
  Contains wheat flour.

⚠ **Post Honeycomb**
25 g Net Carbs per 1⅓ cups
  Contains added sugars.

⚠ **Post 100% Bran**
16 g Net Carbs per ⅓ cup
  Contains added sugars.

HOT CEREAL

Whole grains are among the last foods you'll add back to your eating plan on Atkins, due to their relatively high carb count. Because of this, you will be consuming them in smaller portions and less frequently.

If you are in Induction, enjoy controlled-carb hot cereal with half-and-half diluted with water, unsweetened soymilk, or Atkins-Approved Hood Carb Countdown Dairy Beverage (see page 124) and be sure to calculate in the additional carbs. If you prefer your hot cereal sweet, sprinkle in some Splenda, or drizzle with Atkins Quick Quisine Sugar Free Pancake Syrup. A pinch or two of cinnamon can also contribute some sweetness.

Atkins Hot Cereal, Natural, Sweet Maple, Apple & Cinnamon, Cinnamon & Spice, and Peaches & Cream (Phases 1-4)
3 g Net Carbs per packet

Hodgson Mill Bulgur Wheat with Soy (Phases 3 & 4)
19 g Net Carbs per ¼ cup

Hodgson Mill Multigrain (Phases 3 & 4)
19 g Net Carbs per ⅓ cup

Hodgson Mill Oat Bran (Phases 3 & 4)
17 g Net Carbs per ¼ cup

McCann's Irish Oat Bran (Phases 3 & 4)
11 g Net Carbs per ¼ cup

McCann's Irish Oatmeal, Steel Cut (Phases 3 & 4)
22 g Net Carbs per ¼ cup

McCann's Quick-Cooking Irish Oatmeal (Phases 3 & 4)
22 g Net Carbs per ½ cup

Mother's Oat Bran (Phases 3 & 4)
18 g Net Carbs per ½ cup

Nabisco Cream of Wheat (Phases 3 & 4)
24 g Net Carbs per 3 tablespoons

Old Wessex Instant Wholegrain Oatmeal (Phases 3 & 4)
23 g Net Carbs per ½ cup

Quaker Instant Oatmeal (Phases 3 & 4)
16 g Net Carbs per packet

Quaker Multigrain (Phases 3 & 4)
24 g Net Carbs per ½ cup

Quaker Oat Bran (Phases 3 & 4)
19 g Net Carbs per ½ cup

Quaker Old-Fashioned Oats, Quick (Phases 3 & 4)
23 g Net Carbs per ½ cup

Quaker Grits, Quick (Phases 3 & 4)
27 g Net Carbs per ¼ cup

Wheatena (Phases 3 & 4)
27 g Net Carbs per ⅓ cup

SOME LIKE IT HOT

What is more comforting on a cold winter morning than an old-fashioned bowl of hot cereal? If you're in the later phases of Atkins and your ACE is high enough (see page 14), you can enjoy a bowl of whole-grain, old-fashioned oatmeal. Oats are one of the most nutritious grains, because the hull and germ are not removed when they are rolled or processed. Dress up your oatmeal with a tablespoon or two of nuts, heavy cream, butter, or controlled-carb syrup. Also try hot flax meal mixed with ricotta cheese—it tastes just like creamy, hot cereal.

WHEAT GERM AND BRAN

High in fiber, vitamin E, and a host of other vitamins and minerals, wheat germ (the inner kernel of the grain) and bran (the outer coating) can add nutrients and crunch to several dishes. Sprinkle a couple of tablespoons over plain yogurt, use as a coating for fish or chicken, or sprinkle into your favorite meatloaf recipe in lieu of bread crumbs or cracker crumbs.

Hodgson Mill Untoasted Wheat Germ (Phases 1-4)
3 g Net Carbs per 2 tablespoons

Hodgson Mill Wheat Bran (Phases 1-4)
3 g Net Carbs per 2 tablespoons

Kretschmer Original Wheat Germ (Phases 1-4)
4 g Net Carbs per 2 tablespoons

Quaker Unprocessed Bran (Phases 1-4)
3 g Net Carbs per 2 tablespoons

➤ BREAKFAST AND GRANOLA BARS ◄

You can't beat the convenience of a bar for a fast, nutritious breakfast. Unfortunately, granola bars—once considered the quintessential health food—are often held together with honey or corn syrup. That fact, on top of the grains themselves, means that finding a low-carb selection is like finding a needle in a haystack! Think of these more as grain-based candy bars, not health food, and pass them by or choose a controlled-carb breakfast or nutrition bar instead. (See page 250 for nutrition bars.)

Atkins Morning Start Breakfast Bars, Creamy Cinnamon Bun, Blueberry Muffin, Chocolate Chip Crisp, Apple Crisp (Phases 1-4)
2 g Net Carbs per bar

FYI **Carborite Cereal Bars, Blueberry, Strawberry, Cinnamon Bun (Phases 1-4)**
4 g Net Carbs per bar
Contains enriched wheat flour.

⚠ **Health Valley Moist & Chewy Peanut Crunch**
17 g Net Carbs per bar
Contains added sugars.

⚠ **Health Valley Moist & Chewy Dutch Apple**
20 g Net Carbs per bar
Contains added sugars.

⚠ **Health Valley Cereal Barn Blueberry Cobbler**
26 g Net Carbs per bar
Contains added sugars.

⚠ **Nature Valley Chewy with Yogurt, Blueberry, Strawberry, Vanilla**
25 g Net Carbs per bar
Contains added sugars.

⚠ **Nature Valley Crunchy Cinnamon, Oats 'n Honey, Peanut Butter**
27 g Net Carbs per 2 bars
Contains added sugars.

⚠ **Nutri-Grain Cereal Bars, Apple, Blueberry, Cherry, Mixed Berry, Raspberry, Strawberry**
26 g Net Carbs per bar
Contains added sugars.

⚠ **Nutri-Grain Chewy Granola Bars, Chocolatey Chip, Honey Oat & Raisin, Mixed Berry**
21 g Net Carbs per bar
Contains added sugars.

⚠ **Quaker Fruit & Oatmeal Bars, most flavors**
17 g Net Carbs per bar
   Contains added sugars.

➤ MUFFINS ◄

   When it comes to ready-to-eat muffins, there's still very little out there when you're watching carbs. Seek out controlled-carb versions from companies specializing in controlled-carb food products, as well as those from local bakeries. Controlled-carb muffin mixes offer up more options. (See page 162 for muffin mixes.)

FYI **Atkins Morning Start Ready-to-Eat Muffins, Banana Nut, Corn, Blueberry (Phases 1-4)**
<6 g Net Carbs per muffin, varies by flavor
   Contains enriched wheat flour.

⚠ **Vitamuffin, Multibran, Cran Bran**
20 g Net Carbs per muffin
   Contains added sugars.

WORST BITES: Between the grains and the dried fruits, Uncle Ben's Seven Grain Cereal & Fruit is a carb catastrophe: One bowl supplies a jaw-dropping 69 grams of Net Carbs. And if you're setting down bowls filled with healthier-sounding Apple Jacks cereal or Kix for your little ones, it's time to rethink what you're giving them for that most important meal of the day: They contain 30 grams of Net Carbs and 0 grams of fiber per cup, and 25 grams of Net Carbs and 1 gram of fiber per 1⅓ cups, respectively.

GOT MILK?

As if the Net Carbs counts for most cereals weren't high enough, they climb even *higher* when you add milk. One cup of whole milk ups the total grams of Net Carbs by 11 grams. Milk is okay in moderation in Pre-Maintenance and Lifetime Maintenance, but a carb-rich breakfast can send your blood sugar soaring, and then bring it crashing well before lunchtime. At that point you'll be hungry and irritable—and all too ready to eat whatever food is most convenient, not the smartest choice. Fortunately, these days, there are other controlled-carb options to pour over cereal or stir into decaffeinated hot beverages (see page 123):

- Atkins-Approved Hood Carb Countdown Dairy Beverage (3 g Net Carbs per cup)
- Soymilk, unsweetened
  (1-5 g Net Carbs per cup, varies by brand)
- Heavy cream or half-and-half, mixed with water
  (2.5 g Net Carbs, using ½ cup cream and ½ cup water)

The Breads Aisle

Until recently, the bread aisle was in short supply of acceptable choices for anyone following a controlled-carb lifestyle. But these days there is a growing array of tasty and versatile options, including Atkins Bakery sliced bread and bagels and other Atkins-approved products. You can even enjoy a slice of Atkins Bakery Ready-to-Eat Sliced Bread in your daily meal plan during Induction. That's incredible news for keeping your meals varied and delicious—think open-face sandwiches, eggs and toast, breading for poultry, meat and fish . . . the list goes on.

That said, you have to put a careful eye on the Nutrition Facts panel and ingredients list when you're scouting this area of the supermarket. While we can vouch for Atkins Bakery and Atkins-approved products, a lot of breads contain ingredients that are off-limits on Atkins, such as sugar or sweeteners like honey, molasses or high-fructose corn syrup. You'll also want to steer clear of breads with fruit or cinnamon and other spices swirled into them—like a lot of breads, these often contain artery-clogging hydrogenated oils.

Of course you'll have to consider which phase of Atkins you're in to know which breads are okay for you. As a general guideline, look for breads made with whole grains, and once you're in Pre-Maintenance and Lifetime Maintenance, seek out sandwich-style bread that has no more than 16 grams of Net Carbs per slice—those with 10 or fewer are even better. Some supermarkets are now selling reduced-carb brands of bread and tortillas, which can typically be found in the refrigerator or freezer aisle, or in the in-store bakery section. If your store has a bakery, scope it out for some of the breads listed as well as specialty breads made with 100% whole grains, sprouted grains, or lower-carb flours. (See page 301 for specialty and organic breads.)

And keep an eye on portions, too. For example, The Baker wheat-free loaves are small, but these loaves are dense with whole grains so more than one slice will rack up the carbs.

➤ BREAD PRODUCTS ◄

SANDWICH BREADS

FYI **Atkins Bakery Ready-to-Eat Sliced Bread, Country White, Multigrain, Rye (Phases 1-4)**
3 g Net Carbs per slice
  Contains enriched flour.

FYI **Atkins-Approved Arnold Carb-Counting, Multi-Grain, Whole Wheat (Phases 2-4)**
6 g Net Carbs per slice
  Contains flour.

The Baker Wheat-Free European Linseed (Phases 3 & 4)
13 g Net Carbs per slice

The Baker Wheat-Free Organic Sunflower Seed (Phases 3 & 4)
15 g Net Carbs per slice

⚠ Healthy Home Lower Carb, Italian, White
9 g Net Carbs per slice
  Contains added sugars.

Mestemacher, Fitnessbread, Sunflower Seed Bread (Phases 3 & 4)
16 g Net Carbs per slice

Mestemacher, Pumpernickel (Phases 3 & 4)
17 g Net Carbs per slice

Mestemacher, 3-Grain Bread, Whole Rye Bread (Phases 3 & 4)
18 g Net Carbs per slice

⚠ Sara Lee Delightful Wheat, Delightful White
7 g Net Carbs per slice
　Contains added sugars.

Todd's Organic 3-Carb Bread, Original (Phases 2-4)
1 g Net Carbs per slice

Todd's Organic 4-Carb Bread, Cocoa Breakfast Bread (Phases 2-4)
2 g Net Carbs per slice

⚠ Vermont Bread Company, Alfalfa Sprout, Oat Bran, Oatmeal, Sunflower Sesame, Whole Wheat
12 g Net Carbs per slice
　Contains added sugars.

⚠ Vermont Bread Company Carb Conscious Bread, Wheat, Multigrain
6 g Net Carbs per slice
　Contains added sugars.

⚠ Levy's Rye
16 g Net Carbs per slice
　Contains added sugars and trans fats.

⚠ **Pepperidge Farm Natural Whole Grain, Whole Wheat**
14 g Net Carbs per slice
  Contains added sugars.

Rubschlager Rye-Ola, Pumpernickel, Rye (Phases 3 & 4)
17 g Net Carbs per slice

Rubschlager, Whole Grain (Phases 3 & 4)
11 g Net Carbs per slice

⚠ **Wonder, Whole Wheat**
11 g Net Carbs per slice
  Contains added sugars.

WHY RYE?

Rye is high in fiber. Depending on how much rye flour is used, rye bread may be comparatively low in Net Carbs. But watch out for commercial brands, which may be made with hydrogenated oils.

BAGELS, WRAPS, PITAS, AND ROLLS

  Bagels are often found in the freezer section, while pitas are typically in the bread aisle. Wraps, on the other hand, may be stocked by the deli (tomato, spinach, and herb flavored ones are often here, as are some whole-wheat wraps and specialty flatbreads such as lavash); odds are high that you'll find tortillas in the dairy case (see pages 120–121). If your supermarket doesn't carry controlled-carb brands, the natural foods store may offer more options (see page 308).

FYI **Atkins Bakery Ready-to-Eat Plain Bagels (Phases 2-4)**
7 g Net Carbs per bagel
  Contains enriched flour.

FYI **Atkins Bakery Ready-to-Eat Onion Bagels
(Phases 2-4)**
8 g Net Carbs per bagel
  Contains enriched flour.

FYI **Atkins Bakery Ready-to-Eat Cinnamon-Raisin
Bagels (Phases 2-4)**
9 g Net Carbs per bagel
  Contains enriched flour.

FYI **Atkins Bakery Dinner Rolls (Phases 2-4)**
4 g Net Carbs per roll
  Contains enriched wheat flour.

FYI **Atkins Bakery Sandwich Rolls (Phases 2-4)**
5 g Net Carbs per roll
  Contains enriched wheat flour.

FYI **Atkins Bakery Hot Dog Rolls (Phases 2-4)**
5 g Net Carbs per roll
  Contains enriched wheat flour.

FYI **Atkins Bakery Tortillas (Phases 2-4)**
5 g Net Carbs per tortilla
  Contains enriched flour.

Toufayan Bakeries Low Carb Wraps (Phases 2-4)
7 g Net Carbs per wrap

CYBER TORTILLAS

Can't find controlled-carb or trans fat-free tortillas in your supermarket? Try the 'Net. La Tortilla Factory is one brand that is available from many online retailers, including *www.atkins.com*.

FYI **Thomas' Carb Counting Bagels, White (Phases 3-4)**
18 g Net Carbs per bagel
   Contains flour.

Thomas' Carb Counting Bagels, Whole Wheat (Phases 3 & 4)
16 g Net Carbs per bagel

⚠ **Thomas' Sahara Pita, 100% Whole Wheat**
22 g Net Carbs per pita
   Contains added sugars.

⚠ **Thomas' Sahara Wrap, 100% Whole Wheat**
23 g Net Carbs per wrap
   Contains trans fats and added sugars.

Todd's Organic 2-Carb Bagels, Plain (Phases 1-4)
1 g Net Carbs per ½ bagel

Todd's Organic 4-Carb Rolls (Phases 1-4)
2 g Net Carbs per ½ roll

BREAKING BREAD

Here are some ways to enjoy bread and cut back on carbs:
- Eat only controlled-carb bread.
- Allow yourself only one piece of controlled-carb bread a day during Induction.
- Eat only open-face sandwiches.
- Slice the bread extra thin.
- Eat only the crust.

COCKTAIL BREADS

Cocktail loaves are tiny—often 2–3 inches square and 12–18 inches long, and they're very thinly sliced so the carbs may seem low at first glance. We could not find any brands that did not contain unacceptable ingredients; consider cutting small squares of controlled-carb bread to use as the base for hors d'oeuvres.

⚠️ **Pepperidge Farm Dark Party Bread**
24 g Net Carbs per 5 slices
  Contains trans fats.

⚠️ **Rubschlager Cocktail Bread, Pumpernickel, Rye**
12 g Net Carbs per 3 slices
  Contains added sugars.

BREAD CRUMBS

Avoid the hydrogenated oils and sugars in major brands by making your own bread crumbs. Let slices of controlled-carb bread, such as Atkins Bakery Ready-to-Eat Sliced Bread, dry out or toast them lightly, then whirl them in a food processor. Add dried herbs or other seasonings, if you like. For other options, check out the bread crumbs section in the natural foods section on page 359.

CONTROLLED-CARB COATING MIXES

Many commercial coating mixes, bread crumbs, and stuffings add unnecessary carbs to your meal and often contain hydrogenated oils. Instead of using these, make your own with controlled-carb bread and fresh herbs. Or, for a great alternative, consider this: After the first two weeks of Induction when you can add back nuts, finely ground nuts will add a flavorful and crunchy coating to your chicken and fish. Nuts can burn if exposed to high heat for a long time, so if you do use nuts as a coating, watch the food carefully and adjust the heat as necessary.

⚠ **4C Plain**
20 g Net Carbs per ⅓ cup
  Contains trans fats and sugars.

⚠ **4C Seasoned**
18 g Net Carbs per ⅓ cup
  Contains trans fats and sugars.

⚠ **Progresso, Italian Style**
19 g Net Carbs per ¼ cup
  Contains added sugars.

⚠ **Rienzi, Unseasoned**
24 g Net Carbs per ¼ cup
  Contains added sugars and trans fats.

⚠ **Rienzi, Italian Flavor**
18 g Net Carbs per ¼ cup
  Contains added sugars and trans fats.

⚠ **Ronzoni, Italian Flavor**
21 g Net Carbs per ¼ cup
  Contains added sugars and trans fats.

BRINGING HOME THE BREAD

If you know about flours, you'll have a better idea of which breads to reach for and which to avoid.

- **White, enriched wheat, wheat, bleached, whole wheat:** The first four are refined white flour. Unless the loaf's label specifies "100% whole wheat," there's no telling how much of the whole-grain flour you're getting.

- **100% whole wheat, whole grain, rye, sprouted, sourdough, pumpernickel:** Whole grains, including whole wheat, are lower in carbs and higher in nutrients than refined breads. Rye (including pumpernickel) is too dense to make a palatable bread, so it's often blended with wheat flour. Instead, look for ryes blended with whole-wheat flour.

- **Pumpernickel is not a flour:** A pumpernickel bread has both rye and wheat flour and usually molasses to darken it.

- **Protein:** Protein breads have medium-to-low levels of Net Carbs. What is in them? If they're really full of whole grains they may be stocked in the freezer to maintain freshness.

- **Reduced-carb or low-carb:** These fast-growing categories of breads will be the lowest in Net Carbs, but some manufacturers calculate Net Carbs differently from Atkins—if you don't see the Atkins logo on a product, check the total carbs and the amount of fiber. The actual Net Carbs are total grams of carbs minus grams of fiber (see page 10 in the Introduction).

The Baking Aisle

Sorting the wheat from the chaff is as important in selecting baking products as it is in making them. In order to create remarkably delicious controlled-carb desserts and snacks, you'll have to keep your eye out for compatible ingredients and exciting new products that can make the task easier and more delicious. Some things, like unsweetened cocoa powder and soy flour, are naturally low in carbohydrate; others may be specially formulated items, such as Atkins Quick Quisine Bake Mix.

Refined flour and sugar are very high in carbs. Look for less processed whole-grain flours, such as whole-wheat pastry flour (you may need to head to the natural foods section of your supermarket, or make a special trip to a natural foods store; see page 331). But remember that whole grains are not low in carbs.

Sugar, whether it's the refined white stuff (or its brown cousin) or a so-called healthful sweetener like honey or molasses, should be avoided no matter what phase of Atkins you are in. Added sugars bring nothing to the party but pounds—and dental problems. Splenda, a natural sugar substitute made from sucrose, is our sweetener of choice for baking with excellent results.

➤ BAKING PRODUCTS ◄

MUFFIN, CAKE, COOKIE, AND PANCAKE MIXES

Most of the mainstream commercial bake mixes for cookies, brownies, muffins and cakes are off-limits when you're doing Atkins, thanks not only to high carb counts but unacceptable ingredients like hydrogenated oils and added sugars. Look for the brands we list here; if your store doesn't stock them, ask them to. Most store managers are happy to comply with customer requests.

Atkins Quick Quisine Muffin & Bread Mixes, Blueberry, Corn, Lemon Poppy (Phases 1-4)
3 g Net Carbs per serving

Atkins Quick Quisine Muffin & Bread Mixes, Orange Cranberry, Banana Nut (Phases 1-4)
2 g Net Carbs per serving

Atkins Quick Quisine Muffin & Bread Mix, Chocolate Chocolate Chip (Phases 1-4)
6 g Net Carbs per serving

Atkins Quick Quisine Deluxe Fudge Brownie Mix (Phases 2-4)
9 g Net Carbs per brownie

Atkins Quick Quisine Cookie Mixes, Chocolate Chip, Chocolate Chocolate Chip (Phases 2-4)
6 g Net Carbs per 2 cookies

Atkins Quick Quisine Pancake & Waffle Mixes (Phases 1-4)
3 g Net Carbs per ¼ cup dry mix

Atkins Quick Quisine Deluxe Buttermilk Pancake Mix (Phases 2-4)
8 g Net Carbs per ⅓ cup dry mix

Decadent Desserts Sugar-Free Bake Mix, Almond, Chocolate (Phases 1-4)
0 g Net Carbs per 3 tablespoons mix

⚠ **Hodgson Mill Gingerbread Mix, Whole Wheat**
22 g Net Carbs per ¼ cup mix
   Contains added sugars.

FYI **Hodgson Mill Jalapeño Cornbread Mix (Phases 3 & 4)**
21 g Net Carbs per ¼ cup mix
   Contains flour.

⚠ **No Pudge Fat-Free Brownie Mix, Original, Mint**
21 g Net Carbs per brownie
   Contains added sugars.

⚠ **Sweet'N Low No Sugar Added White Snack Cake Mix**
21 g Net Carbs per ⅓ cup mix
   Contains trans fats.

⚠ **Sweet'N Low No Sugar Added Chocolate Snack Cake Mix**
21 g Net Carbs per ⅓ cup mix
   Contains trans fats.

BAKING CHOCOLATE

Baker's Unsweetened (Phases 1-4)
2 g Net Carbs per ½ square

⚠ **Baker's German Sweet, Semisweet**
7 g Net Carbs per ½ square
   Contains added sugars.

⚠ **Baker's White Chocolate**
8 g Net Carbs per 2 squares
  Contains added sugars.

⚠ **Ghirardelli Semisweet**
22 g Net Carbs per 3 sections
  Contains added sugars.

Ghirardelli Unsweetened (Phases 3 & 4)
7 g Net Carbs per 3 sections

FLAVORING FACTS

Spices, extracts, and seasonings are an excellent way to enhance flavor without adding a lot of carbs. Most spices and extracts provide 0 grams of Net Carbs per serving. Cinnamon, for instance, weighs in with 0.6 grams per teaspoon—the amount you often find per recipe, not per serving.

When it comes to extracts, opt for pure extracts, not artificial ones. You'll be astonished at the difference pure vanilla and pure almond extracts make, compared to their artificial counterparts.

COCOA POWDER, UNSWEETENED

Droste (Phases 1-4)
1 g Net Carbs per tablespoon

Ghirardelli (Phases 1-4)
1 g Net Carbs per tablespoon

Hershey's (Phases 1-4)
2 g Net Carbs per tablespoon

Nestlé (Phases 1-4)
1 g Net Carbs per tablespoon

COCONUT

Skip the sweetened flakes in the baking section and head for the freezer aisle, where you'll find unsweetened coconut, which has a fraction of the Net Carbs as the sweetened stuff and is acceptable in all four phases of Atkins. Natural foods or gourmet stores are a good source for finding unsweetened shredded or grated coconut that has not been frozen—it's delightful whirled into a controlled-carb shake or in later phases as a topping for controlled-carb ice cream.

⚠ Baker's Sweetened Flakes
5 g Net Carbs per 2 tablespoons
  Contains added sugars.

**Torn & Glasser Unsweetened Coconut Flakes
(Phases 1-4)**
3 g Net Carbs per serving

CORNSTARCH

Conventional cornstarch is off-limits on Atkins; therefore the items below earn an Ingredient Alert symbol. Resistant cornstarches, found in controlled-carb baking products, are fine because they do not impact blood sugar. However, when you need to thicken sauces, soups, stews and gravies, ThickenThin Not Starch or Thick-It-Up are ideal all-natural alternatives.

⚠ Argo
7 g Net Carbs per tablespoon

⚠ Hodgson Mill
9 g Net Carbs per 2 teaspoons

Thick-It-Up Thickener (Phases 1-4)
0 g Net Carbs per teaspoon

ThickenThin Not Starch (Phases 1-4)
0 g Net Carbs per teaspoon

EVAPORATED MILK

Evaporated milk has 60% less water than regular milk; it can be used in recipes straight from the can, but if you're using it in lieu of regular milk it must be combined with an equal amount of water. Two conditions when it comes to evaporated milk: First, pass on the low-fat and fat-free varieties; the evaporated milk made from whole milk has less naturally occurring sugar. Second, read the label *carefully* and be sure to choose evaporated—not sweetened condensed—milk, which comes in a similar-looking can.

Most brands (Phases 2-4)
3 g Net Carbs per 2 tablespoons

FLAXSEED

Flaxseed is incredibly rich in omega-3 fatty acids, but your body won't obtain any of the nutritional benefits if you eat the seeds whole—be sure to grind the seeds before you use them. Flaxseeds should be stored in the refrigerator or freezer because they can turn rancid quickly at room temperature.

Hodgson Mill Flaxseed (Phases 1-4)
0 g Net Carbs per 2 tablespoons

FLOUR

It stands to reason that lower-carb foods will contain lower-carb flours. If you're looking for a flour to add crunch or stability to a food before sautéing, reach for soy flour, oat flour, or Atkins Quick Quisine Bake Mix. Note that these cannot be used to replace regular flour in most baking recipes—wheat flour contains gluten, which provides structure to baked goods. For more on flour, see page 331 in the natural foods section.

Atkins Quick Quisine Bake Mix (Phases 1-4)
3 g Net Carbs per ¼ cup dry mix

Arrowhead Mills Oat Flour (Phases 3 & 4)
18 g Net Carbs per ¼ cup

Arrowhead Mills Soy Flour (Phases 1-4)
5 g Net Carbs per ¼ cup

Hodgson Mill Soy Flour (Phases 1-4)
3 g Net Carbs per ¼ cup

Gold Medal Whole-Wheat Flour (Phases 3 & 4)
17 g Net Carbs per ¼ cup

CONTROLLED-CARB FLOUR POWER

Some supermarkets now have a section devoted to controlled-carb foods *(Tip: it may be near the sugar-free foods marketed to diabetics)*. Look for Atkins Quick Quisine Bake Mix here—and pick up a container. Compare its carb count per ¼ cup with that of bleached white flour:
- All-purpose bleached white flour: 23 g Net Carbs
- Atkins Quick Quisine Bake Mix: 3 g Net Carbs

FROSTING

⚠ **Sweet'N Low Chocolate Frosting Mix**
10 g Net Carbs per 2 tablespoons mix
  Contains trans fats.

GELATIN AND PUDDING MIXES

Knox, unflavored (Phases 1-4)
0 g Net Carbs per envelope

Baking Soda, most brands (Phases 1-4)
0-1 g Net Carbs per teaspoon

LEAVENING AGENTS

Fleishmann's Active Dry Yeast (Phases 1-4)
0 g Net Carbs per ¼ teaspoon

SPOTLIGHT ON SUGAR

Sugar masquerades itself under an array of clever names, but as we have said time and time again, your body will never be fooled. Whether it's corn syrup, evaporated cane juice, honey, malt, molasses, fruit juice concentrate, or one of the "oses"—fructose, maltose, dextrose, sucrose, lactose, glucose—it's still sugar. The same is true for sugar in all its colors and forms: From white to brown, turbinado to confectioners', no incarnation of added sugar is acceptable at any phase of Atkins.

SUGAR SUBSTITUTES

Acesulfame Potassium (Ace-K) (Phases 1-4)
<1 g Net Carbs per teaspoon
Ace-K is approximately 200 times sweeter than sugar. Because it cannot be metabolized, it passes through the body without elevating blood sugar. It is sold under the brand name Sunett. Along with sucralose, Ace-K is a sweetener used in some Atkins food products.

Aspartame (Phases 1-4)
1 g Net Carbs per teaspoon
Sold under the brand names Equal and NutraSweet, aspartame cannot be heated, making it unsuitable for cooking or baking.

Saccharin (Phases 1-4)
0.5 g Net Carbs per teaspoon
Although saccharin is allowed on the ANA™, you should limit consumption to no more than three packets per day. Saccharin is sold as Sweet'N Low.

Sucralose (Phases 1-4)
<1 g Net Carbs per teaspoon
Sucralose, which is marketed as Splenda, is the substitute sweetener of choice for anyone doing Atkins. It's the only sugar substitute that's made from sugar, so it tastes like sugar as well as acts like sugar when cooked, but it doesn't perceptibly raise blood sugar. Limit consumption to 3 packets a day.

➤ DRIED FRUITS ◄

You're likely to find dried fruit in the produce aisle, the snack aisle, and the baking aisle as well. But wherever you find it, if you think of dried fruit as a snack, it's time to change your mindset. When fruit is dried, the sugars become concentrated, so it's easy for the carbs to add up after just a few tablespoons of supersweet morsels. So use it to add just a touch of fruity flavor to foods by sprinkling a few pieces on controlled-carb cereal, salads or main dishes. Also, many major brands of dried fruits have been treated with sulfur dioxide, a preservative. Since some people experience an allergic reaction to it, look for those that don't list it in the ingredients. If you can't find sulfur-dioxide-free fruits at the supermarket, check your natural foods store for dried fruits without additives.

APPLES

⚠ Seneca Apple Chips, Original
18 g Net Carbs per 12 chips
  Contains added sugars.

Sun-Maid (Phases 3 & 4)
23 g Net Carbs per ⅓ cup

APRICOTS

If you're inclined to count out the apricots rather than measure or weigh them, pay close attention to whether you're nibbling *whole* dried apricots or dried apricot *halves*; whole apricots will have double the Net Carbs.

Sun-Maid (Phases 3 & 4)
23 g Net Carbs per ¼ cup

Sunsweet (Phases 3 & 4)
20 g Net Carbs per 5 apricots

CHERRIES

⚠ Bentzy's
23 g Net Carbs per ounce
  Contains added sugars.

CRANBERRIES

Because cranberries are so astringent, dried cranberries are almost always loaded with sugar. Read ingredients lists carefully.

⚠ Bentzy's, Plain, with Orange Essence
20 g Net Carbs per ¼ cup
  Contains added sugars.

⚠ Ocean Spray Craisins
31 g Net Carbs per ⅓ cup
  Contains added sugars.

CURRANTS

Dried currants are completely unrelated to the berrylike fresh fruit—they are actually made by drying tiny Champagne grapes. These are also called Corinth grapes, which were corrupted to currant.

Sun-Maid Zante Currants (Phases 3 & 4)
29 g Net Carbs per ¼ cup

DATES, PITTED

Sunsweet (Phases 3 & 4)
29 g Net Carbs per ¼ cup

FIGS

Sun-Maid Orchard Choice (Phases 3 & 4)
23 g Net Carbs per 4 figs

Sun-Maid Calimyrna (Phases 3 & 4)
21 g Net Carbs per ½ cup

Sun-Maid Mission (Phases 3 & 4)
21 g Net Carbs per ¼ cup

FRUIT MIXES

⚠ Sun-Maid, Fruit Bits
27 g Net Carbs per ¼ cup
   Contains added sugars.

⚠ Sun-Maid, Goldens and Cherries
29 g Net Carbs per ¼ cup
   Contains added sugars.

Sun-Maid, Mixed Fruit (Phases 3 & 4)
22 g Net Carbs per ¼ cup

⚠ Sun-Maid, Tropical Medley
31 g Net Carbs per ¼ cup
   Contains added sugars.

Sunsweet, Fruit Morsels (Phases 3 & 4)
28 g Net Carbs per ¼ cup

NECTARINES AND PEACHES

Sun-Maid, California Peaches (Phases 3 & 4)
22 g Net Carbs per ¼ cup

Sunsweet, Dried Nectarines (Phases 3 & 4)
22 g Net Carbs per 3 nectarines

PINEAPPLE AND MANGO

Mariani, Pineapple (Phases 3 & 4)
33 g Net Carbs per ¼ cup

⚠ Sunsweet, Mango
33 g Net Carbs per ⅓ cup
   Contains added sugars.

PRUNES (DRIED PLUMS), PITTED

Sunsweet (Phases 3 & 4)
24 g Net Carbs per 4 prunes

RAISINS

Sun-Maid, Regular and Golden (Phases 3 & 4)
29 g Net Carbs per ¼ cup

SWEETS FOR THE SWEET

As far as sugar substitutes go, sucralose (Splenda) is your best bet. Unlike aspartame (Equal and NutraSweet), it is not metabolized by the body's digestive system, so it passes through quickly without impacting blood sugar levels. It also does not lose its sweetness when heated, so it can be used in cooking and baking with better results than the other sugar substitutes.

Sugar substitutes will satisfy your sweet tooth if you use them wisely. They are powerful sweeteners—most are sweeter than sugar. Except in the case of Splenda, which can be used measure for measure as sugar, you may have to adjust your recipes to use less sugar substitute than regular sugar.

Cooking Tip: To make your own controlled-carb cinnamon-"sugar," mix 1 tablespoon ground cinnamon with ½ cup Splenda.

The Condiments Aisle

Savvy cooks know that the difference between fabulous flavors and "blah" food comes down to condiments. Whether your dish needs the kick of Tabasco, the zest of a Caesar dressing, the tangy bite of mustard, or the salty pungency of olives, condiments add punch—and they usually have modest carb counts.

However, there are a few favorite condiments that will contribute too many carbs in their traditional formulations—regular ketchup, barbecue sauce, teriyaki, marinades, sweet and sour sauce and hoisin sauce, to name a few. In these cases, there are more and more controlled-carb renditions to keep on your radar.

Depending on the size of your supermarket, you may well find condiments in several aisles. The current trend is to organize some by ethnicity, so we've grouped those from Mexican, Asian, and Italian cuisines together. Other condiments—salad dressings, barbecue sauces, and marinades, for example—are organized by brand, so you'll find them listed alphabetically that way within each category.

➤ SALAD DRESSINGS ◄

Whipping up a simple vinaigrette with your favorite oil and vinegar or lemon juice is a snap, and it ensures that your dressing is as low in grams of Net Carbs as possible. Nonetheless, there are times when you want the convenience of a bottled dressing, perhaps with exotic ingredients and flavorings. Always pass by the fat-free and reduced-fat dressings—they're invariably loaded with corn syrup (it has the same consistency as oil and is a cheap substitute). On Atkins, the benefits of healthy fats, such as olive oil, are many: Consuming enough fat helps you stay satisfied, moderates blood sugar and can help control cravings for carbs. When you're controlling carbs, getting adequate dietary fat also accelerates a fat-burning metabolism.

Other red flags in the salad dressing aisle are honey mustards and fruity vinaigrettes—they're almost always high in sugar. Remember, too, that balsamic vinegar contains some sugar and should be limited during Induction.

Atkins Quick Quisine Salad Dressings, "Sweet As Honey" Mustard, Lemon Poppyseed, Country French, Ranch (Phases 1-4)
1 g Net Carbs per 2 tablespoons

⚠️ **Annie's Natural, Balsamic Vinaigrette**
3 g Net Carbs per 2 tablespoons
  Contains added sugars.

Annie's Natural, Caesar, Sea Veggie & Sesame, Shiitake & Sesame (Phases 1-4)
1 g Net Carbs per 2 tablespoons

Annie's Natural, Goddess Dressing, Organic Green Garlic (Phases 1-4)
2 g Net Carbs per 2 tablespoons

Annie's Natural, Tuscany Italian (Phases 2-4)
5 g Net Carbs per 2 tablespoons

FYI **Carb Options, Italian, Ranch (Phases 1-4)**
0 g Net Carbs per 2 tablespoons
  Contains MSG.

Cardini, Lemon Herb, Original Caesar, and Pesto Pasta (Phases 1-4)
1 g Net Carbs per 2 tablespoons

⚠ **Consorzio, Strawberry Balsamic**
2 g Net Carbs per 2 tablespoons
  Contains added sugars.

Drew's Salad Dressing and Marinade, Kalamata Olive & Caper, Roasted Garlic & Peppercorn, Shiitake Ginger, Smoked Tomato, Soy-Ginger (Phases 1-4)
0 g Net Carbs per tablespoon

Drew's Lemon Tahini Goddess Salad Dressing and Marinade (Phases 1-4)
1 g Net Carbs per tablespoon

⚠ **Drew's Salad Dressing and Marinade, Rosemary Balsamic, Thai Sesame Lime, Sesame Orange, Romano Caesar, Garlic Italian**
0-2 g Net Carbs per tablespoon
  Contains added sugars.

Emeril's, Caesar (Phases 1-4)
2 g Net Carbs per 2 tablespoons

Emeril's, House Herb Vinaigrette (Phases 1-4)
1 g Net Carbs per 2 tablespoons

⚠ **Emeril's, Honey Mustard**
3 g Net Carbs per 2 tablespoons
  Contains added sugars.

⚠ **Good Seasons, Italian, Ranch**
1 g Net Carbs per 2 tablespoons
  Contains added sugars.

⚠ **Ken's Steak House, Ranch, Lite Northern Italian**
1 g Net Carbs per 2 tablespoons
  Contains added sugars.

⚠ **Ken's Steak House, Red Wine & Vinegar**
2 g Net Carbs per 2 tablespoons
  Contains added sugars.

⚠ **Ken's Steak House, Olive Oil & Vinaigrette**
0 g Net Carbs per 2 tablespoons
  Contains added sugars.

⚠ **Ken's Steak House, Russian**
5 g Net Carbs per 2 tablespoons
  Contains added sugars.

⚠ **Kraft Seven Seas, Creamy Italian, Red Wine Vinaigrette**
2 g Net Carbs per 2 tablespoons
  Contains added sugars.

⚠ **Kraft Seven Seas, Green Goddess**
1 g Net Carbs per 2 tablespoons
  Contains added sugars.

Maple Grove Farms Low Carb Sugar Free, most flavors (Phases 1-4)
0 g Net Carbs per 2 tablespoons

⚠ **Maple Grove Farms, Lemon 'n Dill**
0 g Net Carbs per 2 tablespoons
  Contains added sugars.

Marie's, Chunky Blue Cheese (Phases 1-4)
0 g Net Carbs per 2 tablespoons

⚠ **Marie's, Creamy Caesar**
2 g Net Carbs per 2 tablespoons
   Contains added sugars.

⚠ **Marie's, Creamy Italian Garlic, Creamy Ranch, Parmesan Ranch**
3 g Net Carbs per 2 tablespoons
   Contains added sugars.

⚠ **Marie's, Chunky Blue Cheese Lite, Chunky Cole Slaw**
6 g Net Carbs per 2 tablespoons
   Contains added sugars.

⚠ **Marie's, Chunky Feta Cheese Dressing**
1 g Net Carbs per 2 tablespoons
   Contains added sugars.

Newman's Own, Olive Oil & Vinegar (Phases 1-4)
1 g Net Carbs per 2 tablespoons

⚠ **Pritikin, Dijon Balsamic Vinaigrette**
6 g Net Carbs per 2 tablespoons
   Contains added sugars.

Walden Farms Calorie Free, all flavors; Sugar Free, all flavors (Phases 1-4)
0 g Net Carbs per 2 tablespoons

OILS AND VINEGARS

As long as you stick with unflavored oils and vinegars, you can be assured that your oil will be free of carbs and your vinegar will be quite low. Add fruits, vegetables, and even some herbs, though, and you may gradually start boosting the grams of Net Carbs.

Keep a variety of oils on hand and look for unrefined, cold-pressed fresh vegetable and nut oils. While they tend to be more expensive, these oils have not been heated and treated with harsh chemicals, which strip away their nutrients, so they still have rich flavor, essential fatty acids and lots of vitamins. Expeller-pressed oils are exposed to heat, however, they retain more of the natural flavor and aroma of the seeds from which they were mechanically pressed than do refined oils. Buy them in small quantities and store them in the fridge.

Oil, unflavored varieties (Phases 1-4)
0 g Net Carbs per tablespoon

Balsamic Vinegar (Phases 2-4)
2-3 g Net Carbs per tablespoon

Cider Vinegar (Phases 1-4)
0 g Net Carbs per tablespoon

Rice Vinegar (Phases 1-4)
0 g Net Carbs per tablespoon

Wine Vinegar (Phases 1-4)
0 g Net Carbs per tablespoon

⚠ Seasoned Rice Vinegar
5 g Net Carbs per tablespoon
  Contains added sugars.

OIL AND VINEGAR HINT

While most oils and vinegars are a safe zero-carb bet, there are some exceptions, primarily those that are flavored and seasoned. If you sprinkle on more than the serving size, you might eat up more carbs than you bargained for. Some examples? Consorzio Roasted Pepper Flavored Olive Oil has 4 grams of Net Carbs per serving. Nakano Seasoned Rice Vinegar also has 4 g Net Carbs per serving.

DIPS

You'll find prepared dips by the chips, in the produce section and in the dairy case (see page 119), and dip mixes by soups and by gravies. Prepared cheese-, buttermilk- (such as ranch) and vegetable-based dips are usually higher in Net Carbs than those that are based on sour cream or mayonnaise. Most major brands also contain unacceptable ingredients like added sugars and hydrogenated oils. Oftentimes, your best bet is combining pure spice blends with sour cream.

Guiltless Gourmet Black Bean Dip, Spicy, Mild (Phases 2-4)
4 g Net Carbs per 2 tablespoons

FYI **Hidden Valley Original Ranch Party (Phases 1-4)**
1 g Net Carbs per ¹⁄₁₆ packet
   Contains MSG.

⚠ Knorr Garden Dill
0 g Net Carbs per ¹⁄₂₀ packet
   Contains trans fats and added sugars.

⚠ **Marie's, Blue Cheese Dip**
2 g Net Carbs per 2 tablespoons
  Contains added sugars and trans fats.

⚠ **Marie's, Dill Dip**
2 g Net Carbs per 2 tablespoons
  Contains added sugars.

⚠ **Marie's, French Onion Dip**
3 g Net Carbs per 2 tablespoons
  Contains added sugars and trans fats.

⚠ **Marzetti Ranch Veggie Dip**
2 g Net Carbs per 2 tablespoons
  Contains added sugars.

Victoria Roasted Red Pepper Dip (Phases 3 & 4)
12 g Net Carbs per ¼ cup

⚠ **Wish-Bone Ranch-Up!**
2 g Net Carbs per 2 tablespoons
  Contains added sugars.

MAYONNAISE

Mayonnaise is made primarily of oil and eggs, but vegetarian versions made with tofu can be found in the natural foods section of most supermarkets. All major brands of regular mayonnaise contain small amounts of added sugar; reduced-fat, light, and fat-free versions contain even more sugar and other fillers to make up for the flavor and texture provided by oil, making it higher in carbohydrate and less flavorful.

⚠ **Mayonnaise, regular, most brands**
0 g Net Carbs per tablespoon
  Contains added sugars.

Carb Options Whipped Dressing (Phases 1-4)
0 g Net Carbs per tablespoon

Hain (Eggless) (Phases 1-4)
0 g Net Carbs per tablespoon

⚠ **Hellmann's Just 2 Good**
2 g Net Carbs per tablespoon
  Contains added sugars.

⚠ **Hellmann's Light**
1 g Net Carbs per tablespoon
  Contains added sugars.

⚠ **Kraft Fat-Free**
2 g Net Carbs per tablespoon
  Contains added sugars.

⚠ **Kraft Light**
1 g Net Carbs per tablespoon
  Contains added sugars.

⚠ **Miracle Whip Salad Dressing**
2 g Net Carbs per tablespoon
  Contains added sugars.

⚠ **Miracle Whip Salad Dressing Light**
2 g Net Carbs per tablespoon
  Contains added sugars.

⚠️ **Nasoya (soy-based) Nayonaise**
0 g Net Carbs per tablespoon
  Contains added sugars.

⚠️ **Smart Beat**
3 g Net Carbs per tablespoon
  Contains added sugars.

Sugar Busters! Mayonnaise (Phases 1-4)
0 g Net Carbs per tablespoons

TARTAR SAUCE

Tartar sauce is made by combining mayonnaise with vegetables, condiments, like relish, and seasonings, all of which make it higher in Net Carbs. Most brands contain sugar. Prepare your own, using sugar-free mayo, capers and chopped pickle.

⚠️ **Golden Dipt**
3 g Net Carbs per 2 tablespoons
  Contains added sugars.

⚠️ **Gold's**
1 g Net Carbs per teaspoon
  Contains added sugars.

⚠️ **Hellmann's**
3 g Net Carbs per 2 tablespoons
  Contains added sugars.

⚠️ **Kraft**
5 g Net Carbs per 2 tablespoons
  Contains added sugars.

⚠️ **Old Original Bookbinders**
4 g Net Carbs per 2 tablespoons
  Contains added sugars.

➤ MEXICAN CONDIMENTS AND SAUCES ◄

SALSA

Most salsas are tomato-based and seasoned with peppers, garlic, onions, and herbs and spices; others are made with tomatillos. Some brands add sugar and should be avoided. Also, skip those based on fruit, unless they are free of added sugars and you are very near or at your goal weight, and have only a small portion. Don't forget to look in the dairy case for salsa, too (see page 119).

Bravo's, all varieties (Phases 1-4)
3 g Net Carbs per 2 tablespoons

Chi-Chi's Original Recipe, all varieties (Phases 1-4)
2 g Net Carbs per 2 tablespoons

⚠ Coyote Cocina Fire Roasted
1 g Net Carbs per 2 tablespoons
  Contains added sugars.

Coyote Cocina Grilled Garden (Phases 1-4)
3 g Net Carbs per 2 tablespoons

Coyote Cocina New Mexican Green Chile (Phases 1-4)
1 g Net Carbs per 2 tablespoons

**Coyote Cocina Roasted Corn & Black Bean
(Phases 3 & 4)**
1 g Net Carbs per 2 tablespoons

Desert Pepper Salsa Diablo, Salsa Divino (Phases 1-4)
1 g Net Carbs per 2 tablespoons

Frontera, Habanero, Jalapeño Cilantro (Phases 1-4)
2 g Net Carbs per 2 tablespoons

Frontera, Roasted Poblano (Phases 1-4)
3 g Net Carbs per 2 tablespoons

⚠ **Frontera, Roasted Tomato, Roasted Red Pepper and Garlic, Tomatillo, Rustic Guajillo**
3 g Net Carbs per 2 tablespoons
  Contains added sugars.

Muir Glen Organic Black Bean & Corn (Phases 3 & 4)
2 g Net Carbs per 2 tablespoons

Muir Glen Organic Salsa, Mild, Medium, Garlic Cilantro (Phases 1-4)
2 g Net Carbs per 2 tablespoons

Newman's Own Bandito, Mild (Phases 1-4)
2 g Net Carbs per 2 tablespoons

⚠ **Newman's Own Bandito, Medium, Hot**
2 g Net Carbs per 2 tablespoons
  Contains added sugars.

⚠ **Newman's Own Chunky Pineapple**
2 g Net Carbs per 2 tablespoons
  Contains added sugars.

⚠ **Newman's Own Roasted Garlic**
2 g Net Carbs per 2 tablespoons
  Contains added sugars.

⚠ **Old El Paso Thick 'n Chunky, Mild, Medium**
3 g Net Carbs per 2 tablespoons
  Contains added sugars.

FYI **Taco Bell, Salsa con Queso (Phases 1-4)**
2 g Net Carbs per 2 tablespoons
  Contains MSG.

⚠️ **Taco Bell, Thick 'n Chunky**
2 g Net Carbs per 2 tablespoons
   Contains added sugars.

Walnut Acres Organic, Fiesta Cilantro (Phases 1-4)
2 g Net Carbs per 2 tablespoons

Walnut Acres Organic, Midnight Sun (Phases 3 & 4)
3 g Net Carbs per 2 tablespoons

⚠️ **Walnut Acres Organic Sweet Southwestern Peach**
5 g Net Carbs per 2 tablespoons
   Contains added sugars.

ENCHILADA SAUCE

⚠️ **Old El Paso**
3 g Net Carbs per ¼ cup
   Contains added sugars.

La Victoria, Traditional (Phases 1-4)
2 g Net Carbs per ¼ cup

TACO SAUCE

La Victoria, Red (Phases 1-4)
1 g Net Carbs per tablespoon

⚠️ **Old El Paso**
1 g Net Carbs per tablespoon
   Contains added sugars.

⚠️ **Ortega**
2 g Net Carbs per tablespoon
   Contains added sugars.

⚠ **Taco Bell**
2 g Net Carbs per tablespoon
Contains added sugars.

JALAPEÑOS

B&G (Phases 1-4)
1 g Net Carbs per ounce (about 2 peppers)

La Victoria (Phases 1-4)
2 g Net Carbs per 1½ tablespoons

Old El Paso (Phases 1-4)
2 g Net Carbs per 2 tablespoons

➤ ASIAN CONDIMENTS AND SAUCES ◄

BLACK BEAN SAUCE

Ka-Me (Phases 1-4)
3 g Net Carbs per tablespoon

⚠ **Kikkoman**
4 g Net Carbs per 2 tablespoons
Contains added sugars.

⚠ **Roland**
7 g Net Carbs per 2 tablespoons
Contains added sugars.

HOISIN SAUCE

Hoisin is a thick, tangy sauce made of fermented soybeans. Check the ingredients list—most brands list sugar, syrup, or water as the first ingredient. Keep looking until you find a brand with soybeans listed first—and no added sugar. Steel's Gourmet is one acceptable brand available at many natural foods stores (see page 359).

⚠ House of Tsang
4 g Net Carbs per 2 tablespoons
  Contains added sugars.

⚠ Ka-Me
15 g Net Carbs per 2 tablespoons
  Contains added sugars.

⚠ Kikkoman
17 g Net Carbs per 2 tablespoons
  Contains added sugars.

⚠ Roland
10 g Net Carbs per tablespoon
  Contains added sugars.

SOY SAUCE

Soy sauce can be made with soybeans, wheat, or barley; the key to choosing a top-quality soy sauce is to look for the word "fermented" on the label. Other soy sauces are chemically processed and have an unpleasant, harsh taste. Soy sauce is extremely high in sodium, though "lite" varieties contain somewhat less. During Induction and OWL, sodium is less of a concern for people who are not salt-sensitive—you may salt (or use soy sauce) to taste in order to avoid electrolyte loss. Tamari is a Japanese soy sauce; it is similar to Chinese sauces. Be wary of added sweeteners, like molasses, in soy sauce.

Kikkoman (Phases 1-4)
0 g Net Carbs per tablespoon

Kikkoman Lite (Phases 1-4)
1 g Net Carbs per tablespoon

⚠️ La Choy
1 g Net Carbs per tablespoon
Contains added sugars.

⚠️ La Choy Lite
2 g Net Carbs per tablespoon
Contains added sugars.

San-J Premium Tamari Soy Sauce (Phases 1-4)
1 g Net Carbs per tablespoon

TERIYAKI SAUCE

Atkins Quick Quisine Teriyaki Sauce (Phases 1-4)
1 g Net Carbs per tablespoon

Carb Options (Phases 1-4)
1 g Net Carbs per tablespoon

⚠️ San-J Teriyaki Sauce
3 g Net Carbs per tablespoon
Contains added sugars.

FISH SAUCE

Common in Thailand (where it's called *nam pla*) and Vietnam (where it's called *nuoc nam*), fish sauce is a pungent, salty condiment made from fermented fish. Major brands contain added sugars.

⚠️ Roland
1 g Net Carbs per tablespoon
Contains added sugars.

⚠ A Taste of Thai
1 g Net Carbs per tablespoon
Contains added sugars.

⚠ Thai Kitchen
3 g Net Carbs per tablespoon
Contains added sugars.

SWEET & SOUR SAUCE

You'll be hard-pressed to find a low-carb, low-sugar sweet & sour sauce in your supermarket. Steel's Gourmet Sweet & Sour Sauce with 2 grams of Net Carbs is available at most natural foods stores (see page 359).

⚠ Kraft
13 g Net Carbs per tablespoon
Contains added sugars.

⚠ San-J Sweet & Tangy Sauce
13 g Net Carbs per tablespoon
Contains added sugars.

⚠ World Harbors Maui Mountain Hawaiian Style
14 g Net Carbs per tablespoon
Contains added sugars.

WASABI

You'll find wasabi paste (the green condiment served alongside pickled ginger with sushi) in tubes; wasabi powder comes in small glass jars. This fiery Japanese condiment is made from horseradish.

Most brands (Phases 1-4)
0 g Net Carbs per teaspoon

BABY CORN

Baby corns are the miniature corn cobs often found in Asian stir-fries. While they look like tiny ears of corn, they taste less sweet—and have fewer carbs.

⚠ Asian Gourmet
1 g Net Carbs per 3 pieces
  Contains added sugars.

Roland (Phases 3 & 4)
2 g Net Carbs per ½ cup

Season (Phases 3 & 4)
1 g Net Carbs per ½ cup

BAMBOO SHOOTS

Asian Gourmet (Phases 1-4)
0 g Net Carbs per ½ cup

Geisha (Phases 1-4)
1 g Net Carbs per ½ cup

La Choy (Phases 1-4)
2 g Net Carbs per ½ cup

Roland (Phases 1-4)
1 g Net Carbs per ½ cup

WATER CHESTNUTS

Roland, whole (Phases 2-4)
8 g Net Carbs per ½ cup

Season, sliced (Phases 2-4)
8 g Net Carbs per ½ cup

➤ ITALIAN AND MEDITERRANEAN ◄
CONDIMENTS AND SAUCES

ANCHOVIES AND ANCHOVY PASTE

If you use only a few anchovies at a time, look for resealable glass jars. You might find anchovies packed in salt in Italian markets; they should be rinsed. Oil-packed anchovies should be drained. Anchovy paste is a wonderful way to add flavor to dressings and many recipes.

Anchovies, most brands (Phases 1-4)
0 g Net Carbs per fillet

Jean Gui Anchovy Paste (Phases 1-4)
0 g Net Carbs per tablespoon

Roland Anchovy Paste (Phases 1-4)
0 g Net Carbs per tablespoon

ARTICHOKE HEARTS

Marinated artichoke hearts are wonderful for tossing into salads or with controlled-carb pasta. Be aware that some artichoke hearts contain partially hydrogenated oils—read ingredients lists with care.

Cento (Phases 1-4)
2 g Net Carbs per 2 pieces

Roland (Phases 1-4)
1 g Net Carbs per 2 pieces

⚠ Season
2 g Net Carbs per ounce
Contains trans fats.

CAPERS

Made by pickling buds from a shrub native to the Mediterranean, capers come in two sizes: the smaller French nonpareils and larger Italian capers. Most often you'll find capers in brine, but specialty markets may sell salt-packed capers. Both should be rinsed before using.

Most national brands (Phases 1-4)
1 g Net Carbs per tablespoon

OLIVES AND OLIVE PASTE

Look for olive bars in the produce section. If your market doesn't have one, stick with olives in jars, not cans—their flavor is much better. Olives are a fantastic source of mono-unsaturated fats and a great snack even on Induction, when you can have 10–20 per day. Olive paste adds zip to sandwiches prepared on controlled-carb bread.

Olives, most national brands, all varieties, including stuffed with pimientos (Phases 1-4)
0-1 g Net Carbs per 5 olives

Bel Aria Black Olive Paste (Phases 1-4)
2 g Net Carbs per 2 tablespoons

EGGPLANT APPETIZERS

Caponata, or Sicilian eggplant appetizer, can be found in jars near Italian condiments. Toss some with controlled-carb pasta for a fast dinner.

Progresso (Phases 1-4)
0 g Net Carbs per 2 tablespoons

HEARTS OF PALM

Roland (Phases 1-4)
2 g Net Carbs per ½ cup

Season (Phases 1-4)
1 g Net Carbs per ½ cup

ROASTED RED PEPPERS/PIMIENTOS

B&G (Phases 1-4)
0 g Net Carbs per ounce (about 2 peppers)

Mancini (Phases 1-4)
2 g Net Carbs per ounce (about 2 peppers)

Roland (Phases 1-4)
4 g Net Carbs per ounce (about 2 peppers)

SUN-DRIED TOMATOES (IN OLIVE OIL)

Roland (Phases 1-4)
2 g Net Carbs per 2 pieces

Sonoma (Phases 1-4)
2 g Net Carbs per 2-3 halves

TAHINI

Made by grinding sesame seeds into a paste, tahini has a slightly sweet flavor.

Arrowhead Mills (Phases 2-4)
1 g Net Carbs per 2 tablespoons

Joyva (Phases 2-4)
2 g Net Carbs per 2 tablespoons

SNACK FACTS

Looking for a nice nibble or a post-lunch munch? Try vegetable-based snacks. Olives, artichoke hearts, dill pickles, hearts of palm, and avocados provide the boost you need with a minimum number of Net Carbs. Here's the skinny:
- 0.7 g Net Carbs per 5 black olives
- 2.5 g Net Carbs per 5 green olives
- 1 g Net Carbs per 6 artichoke hearts
- 1 g Net Carbs per ½ cup hearts of palm
- 2 g Net Carbs per whole kosher dill pickle

➤ BARBECUE SAUCE ◄

Sweet and smoky, most barbecue sauce is chock-full of sugar, molasses or corn syrup, making it high in carbohydrate. Look for low-carb lines.

Atkins Quick Quisine Barbeque Sauce (Phases 1-4)
1 g Net Carbs per tablespoon

⚠ Annie's Natural, Original Recipe BBQ Sauce
9 g Net Carbs per 2 tablespoons
Contains added sugars.

⚠ Bull's-Eye, Original
13 g Net Carbs per tablespoon
Contains added sugars.

Carb Options Barbecue Sauce, Hickory (Phases 1-4)
3 g Net Carbs per 2 tablespoons

⚠️ **Carb Options Barbecue Sauce, Original**
3 g Net Carbs per 2 tablespoons
   Contains added sugars.

⚠️ **Jack Daniel's Original No. 7**
12 g Net Carbs per tablespoon
   Contains added sugars.

⚠️ **KC Masterpiece, Original**
15 g Net Carbs per 2 tablespoons
   Contains added sugars.

⚠️ **Kraft, Original**
9 g Net Carbs per tablespoon
   Contains added sugars.

⚠️ **Open Pit, Original**
11 g Net Carbs per tablespoon
   Contains added sugars.

⚠️ **Stubb's, Mild**
6 g Net Carbs per tablespoon
   Contains added sugars.

Walden Farms Barbeque Sauce (Phases 1-4)
0 g Net Carbs per tablespoon

➤ OTHER CONDIMENTS ◄

KETCHUP

Do you know what a tablespoon of ketchup looks like? If you generally pour it out with no thought to measure, squeeze some into a measuring spoon then put it on your plate. How does it compare to what you normally eat? Most ketchup is full of sugar, so opt for one of the unsweetened or controlled-carb brands on the market.

Atkins Quick Quisine Ketch-a-Tomato (Phases 1-4)
1 g Net Carbs per tablespoon

⚠ Heinz
4 g Net Carbs per tablespoon
  Contains added sugars.

Heinz Low-Carb Ketchup (Phases 1-4)
1 g Net Carbs per tablespoon

⚠ Hunt's
4 g Net Carbs per tablespoon
  Contains added sugars.

Walden Farms (Phases 1-4)
0 g Net Carbs per tablespoon

Westbrae Unsweetened Un-Ketchup (Phases 1-4)
1 g Net Carbs per tablespoon

MARINADES

The simplest marinades include oil, an acid (such as vinegar or lemon juice) and seasonings. Watch out for those that contain sugar or corn syrup.

⚠ A.1. Marinade, Classic
3 g Net Carbs per tablespoon
  Contains added sugars.

⚠ Adolph's Marinades in Minutes Garlic, Original Chicken, Original Meat
1 g Net Carbs per ¾ teaspoon
  Contains added sugars.

⚠ Adolph's Marinades in Minutes Original Meat Sodium Free
2 g Net Carbs per ¼ teaspoon
　Contains added sugars.

⚠ Annie's Natural Organic, Smoky Campfire
1 g Net Carbs per tablespoon
　Contains added sugars.

⚠ Annie's Natural Organic, Spicy Ginger
3 g Net Carbs per tablespoon
　Contains added sugars.

⚠ Consorzio, Baja Lime, Tropical Grill
3 g Net Carbs per tablespoon
　Contains added sugars.

⚠ Consorzio, Lemon Pepper
1 g Net Carbs per tablespoon
　Contains added sugars.

Emeril's, Lemon, Rosemary & Gaaahlic (Phases 1-4)
1 g Net Carbs per tablespoon

⚠ Emeril's, Roasted Vegetable
1 g Net Carbs per tablespoon
　Contains added sugar.

Golden Dipt, Lemon Herb (Phases 1-4)
0 g Net Carbs per tablespoon

⚠ Golden Dipt, White Wine Dijon
1 g Net Carbs per tablespoon
　Contains added sugars.

⚠ **Kikkoman Teriyaki Marinade & Sauce**
2 g Net Carbs per tablespoon
 Contains added sugars.

⚠ **Lawry's 30 Minute Marinade Mesquite**
1 g Net Carbs per tablespoon
 Contains added sugars.

⚠ **McCormick Meat Marinade Mix, Fajitas**
3 g Net Carbs per 2 teaspoons dry mix
 Contains added sugars.

⚠ **McCormick Meat Marinade Mix, Meat**
2 g Net Carbs per 2 teaspoons dry mix
 Contains added sugars.

⚠ **McCormick Grill Mates Marinade, Southwest, Zesty Herb**
1 g Net Carbs per 2 teaspoons
 Contains added sugars.

STEAK SAUCE

Atkins Quick Quisine Steak Sauce (Phases 1-4)
1 g Net Carbs per tablespoon

⚠ **A.1., Original**
3 g Net Carbs per tablespoon
 Contains added sugars.

⚠ **Carb Options Steak Sauce**
1 g Net Carbs per tablespoon
 Contains added sugars.

⚠ **Heinz 57**
4 g Net Carbs per tablespoon
  Contains added sugars.

⚠ **Lea & Perrins**
5 g Net Carbs per tablespoon
  Contains added sugars.

⚠ **Newman's Own**
4 g Net Carbs per tablespoon
  Contains added sugars.

Pickapeppa Sauce (Phases 1-4)
1 g Net Carbs per teaspoon

HOT SAUCE

Most brands (Phases 1-4)
0 g Net Carbs per teaspoon

Tabasco (Phases 1-4)
0 g Net Carbs per teaspoon

CLAM JUICE

Most brands (Phases 1-4)
0 g Net Carbs per cup

GRAVY (JARRED AND CANNED)

Prepared gravy almost always contains flour, cornstarch and/or sugars.

⚠ **Franco-American Beef Gravy**
3 g Net Carbs per ¼ cup
  Contains added sugars.

MUSTARD

You'll find an enormous array of mustards in some super-markets (and even more in specialty stores and gourmet markets). Steer clear of sweet mustards, whether they're made with honey, brown sugar, or are simply labeled "sweet-hot."

Chinese-Style (Phases 1-4)
1 g Net Carbs per teaspoon

Dijon (Phases 1-4)
0 g Net Carbs per teaspoon

⚠ Honey-Mustard
2 g Net Carbs per teaspoon
   Contains added sugars.

Yellow (Phases 1-4)
0 g Net Carbs per teaspoon

BACON BITS

While regular bacon is okay on Atkins, even real pack-aged bacon bits can be swimming in hydrogenated oils. Check labels carefully, and if you can't find any that are ac-ceptable, crumble up some crisp-cooked real bacon.

⚠ Hormel Real Bacon Bits
0 g Net Carbs per tablespoon
   Contains added sugars.

⚠ McCormick Bacon 'n Pieces
2 g Net Carbs per tablespoon
   Contains trans fats.

⚠ **Spice Supreme Imitation Bacon Bits**
2 g Net Carbs per tablespoon
  Contains trans fats.

COCKTAIL ONIONS

Most brands (Phases 1-4)
0 g Net Carbs per 10 pieces

HORSERADISH

Gold's (Phases 1-4)
0 g Net Carbs per teaspoon

⚠ **Inglehoffer**
0 g Net Carbs per teaspoon
  Contains added sugars.

HOT CHERRY PEPPERS

Most brands (Phases 1-4)
2 g Net Carbs per ounce (about 2 peppers)

CHIPOTLE EN ADOBO

Chile Today (Phases 1-4)
2 g Net Carbs per 2 peppers

PICKLES

Sour pickles and kosher dills are your best bets. Bread-and-butter chips, half-sour, and sweet pickles usually contain added sugars and should be avoided.

⚠ **B&G Bread & Butter Chips**
7 g Net Carbs per 6 pieces
  Contains added sugars.

B&G Kosher Dills (Phases 1-4)
0 g Net Carbs per ½ pickle

⚠ **B&G Sweet Gherkins**
9 g Net Carbs per 4½ pickles
Contains added sugars.

⚠ **Claussen Bread & Butter Chips**
4 g Net Carbs per 6 pieces
Contains added sugars.

Claussen Kosher Dills (Phases 1-4)
1 g Net Carbs per ½ pickle

⚠ **Heinz Sweet Gherkins**
7 g Net Carbs per 2 pickles
Contains added sugars.

⚠ **Vlasic Bread & Butter Chips**
7 g Net Carbs per 3 chips
Contains added sugars.

Vlasic Kosher Dills (Phases 1-4)
1 g Net Carbs per ½ pickle

⚠ **Vlasic Sweet Gherkins**
9 g Net Carbs per 3 pickles
Contains added sugars.

SWEET RELISH

⚠ **B&G**
4 g Net Carbs per tablespoon
Contains added sugars.

⚠️ **Vlasic**
4 g Net Carbs per tablespoon
  Contains added sugars.

HOT DOG RELISH

⚠️ **B&G**
5 g Net Carbs per tablespoon
  Contains added sugars.

⚠️ **Vlasic**
4 g Net Carbs per tablespoon
  Contains added sugars.

SAUERKRAUT

Look for sauerkraut in jars rather than cans, or check the meat department for bagged sauerkraut.

B&G (Phases 1-4)
1 g Net Carbs per 2 tablespoons

Hebrew National (Phases 1-4)
0 g Net Carbs per 2 tablespoons

JAMS, JELLIES, AND PRESERVES

Combine no-sugar-added jams (try raspberry or apricot) with mustard or vinegar for tangy, controlled-carb basting sauces—you'll need a tablespoon or so of both, and the mixture will be enough to cover a whole pork tenderloin or roast chicken.

For the truest flavor, avoid so-called "all-fruit" spreads. They're sweetened with grape or other juices, which can dilute the taste of the preserved fruit—and add more sugar. Look for

Steel's Gourmet Jams in your natural foods store. (See page 358 for more options.)

▲ **Cascadian Farm Fruit Spread, all flavors**
10 g Net Carbs per tablespoon
  Contains added sugars.

▲ **Polaner All Fruit Spreadable Fruit, all flavors**
10 g Net Carbs per tablespoon
  Contains added sugars.

Polaner All Fruit Sugar-Free Jam, Apricot, Seedless Raspberry, Strawberry (Phases 3 & 4)
5 g Net Carbs per tablespoon

FYI **Smucker's Light Preserves, Apricot, Boysenberry, Grape, Orange, Red Raspberry, Seedless Blackberry, Strawberry (Phases 3 & 4)**
5 g Net Carbs per tablespoon
  Contains aspartame.

▲ **Smucker's Low-Sugar Preserves, all flavors**
6 g Net Carbs per tablespoon
  Contains added sugars.

WE'RE JAMMIN'

How much no-sugar-added jam should you spread on your bread? A serving is 1 tablespoon—all you need for plenty of fruit flavor without tons of carbs.

SUGAR: WHAT'S IN A NAME?

When you're doing Atkins, you're already scanning ingredients labels for words that mean sugar, such as brown syrup, evaporated cane juice, glucose, dextrose and corn syrup. Keep an eye out for the following terms too: They can help you get a better handle on what's sweet—and what can sour your weight-loss efforts.

Sugar-free or sugar-less: The term "free" means that a product contains no amount of, or only trivial amounts of, an ingredient, such as fat, saturated fat, cholesterol, sodium, sugars, and calories. "Sugar-free" indicates that the product contains less than 0.5 grams of sugars per serving.

No sugar added, without added sugar, no added sugar: Products that bear these labels contain no sugar or ingredients, like fruit juice, which can be substituted for sugar. In addition, they do not contain ingredients made with added sugars, such as jam or concentrated fruit juice.

Naturally occurring sugar: You won't see this term on a package, but a product containing naturally occurring sugars includes sugars found in foods in their natural state. For example, fruit sugar, or fructose, naturally occurs in apples and other fruits; lactose, or milk sugar, naturally occurs in milk and other dairy products. Vegetables also contain natural sugars. Natural sugars, in moderation, are fine on Atkins—just remember to tally the carbs provided by these items into your daily carb intake. Unfortunately, the Nutrition Facts panel doesn't differentiate between "naturally occurring sugars" and added sugars. But you can tell the difference by checking the list of ingredients—only added sugars will be listed on the label.

Tap 'n Apple Apple Butter Spread (Phases 3 & 4)
4 g Net Carbs per tablespoon

PANCAKE AND FLAVORED SYRUPS

Real maple syrup is absolutely loaded with carbs—13 grams per measly tablespoon, to be exact. Check your natural foods store for more controlled-carb brands. Use Atkins Sugar Free Flavored Syrups to flavor plain seltzer or drizzle some over your favorite controlled-carb dessert.

Atkins Quick Quisine Pancake Syrup (Phases 1-4)
0 g Net Carbs per 2 ounces

Atkins Sugar Free Flavored Syrups, Caramel, Chocolate, Raspberry, Strawberry, Hazelnut, Vanilla, Cola, Lemon Lime, Ginger Ale, Root Beer (Phases 1-4)
0 g Net Carbs per tablespoon

FYI Cary's Sugar-Free (Phases 1-4)
1 g Net Carbs per ¼ cup
Contains aspartame.

Log Cabin Sugar-Free (Phases 1-4)
0 g Net Carbs per ¼ cup

Maple Grove Farms Sugar-Free (Phases 1-4)
1 g Net Carbs per ¼ cup

Smucker's Sugar-Free Breakfast Syrup (Phases 1-4)
1 g Net Carbs per ¼ cup

WORCESTERSHIRE SAUCE

 Most brands
1 g Net Carbs per teaspoon
   Contains added sugars.

PANCAKE SYRUP: CARBS IN A BOTTLE

Whether you pour it on pancakes or mix it into a basting sauce for ham, be sure to use sugar-free pancake syrup. Take a look at these numbers:
   - Sugar-free pancake syrup,   *0–1 g Net Carbs*
     most brands   *per ¼ cup*
   - Light pancake syrup,   *24–26 g Net Carbs*
     most brands   *per ¼ cup*
   - Pure maple syrup,   *52–55 g Net Carbs*
     most brands   *per ¼ cup*

The Canned and Jarred Foods Aisle

True or false: Canned foods are nutritionally inferior to fresh; canned foods taste too salty; and canned foods—especially vegetables—have a mushy texture?

Canned foods do tend to be salty, and their texture can vary considerably from one food to another as well as among brands. But some foods are canned just minutes after harvest . . . and some "fresh" foods may have survived a cross-country trucking expedition or have languished in a supermarket's warehouse and be days, if not weeks, from the field.

Canned foods are often more convenient than fresh or from-scratch preparations. Dried beans, for example, must be soaked and then cooked—a process that can take the better part of a day, even using a quick-soak method. Canned meats and fish can be terrific for quick and tasty salads, casseroles, and skillet suppers.

Salt is often added when foods are processed; salt adds flavor, of course, and it acts as a preservative. If you find a food, such as beans, tastes too salty, you can simply rinse them before using; other foods (such as tomatoes) are available in salt-free varieties.

One clear benefit of canned foods: They have Nutrition Facts labels and ingredients lists, so you can be sure of what you're getting.

➤ CANNED AND JARRED PRODUCTS ◄

BEANS AND LEGUMES

Draining off the soaking liquid reduces the sodium and accompanying salty taste of canned beans; rinsing the beans reduces them even further. Introduce beans to your eating plan by tossing a few into a fresh green salad. For more on beans, see pages 235–239.

Adzuki Beans, most brands (Phases 3 & 4)
14 g Net Carbs per ½ cup

Garbanzo Beans, most brands (Phases 3 & 4)
14 g Net Carbs per ½ cup

Black Soybeans, Eden Organic, and most brands (Phases 3 & 4)
1 g Net Carbs per ½ cup

Kidney Beans, most brands (Phases 3 & 4)
12 g Net Carbs per ½ cup

Pinto Beans, most brands (Phases 3 & 4)
12 g Net Carbs per ½ cup

Navy Beans, most brands (Phases 3 & 4)
13 g Net Carbs per ½ cup

Red Lentils, most brands (Phases 3 & 4)
22 g Net Carbs per ¼ cup

Green Split Peas, most brands (Phases 3 & 4)
16 g Net Carbs per ¼ cup

Lentils, most brands (Phases 3 & 4)
10 g Net Carbs per ¼ cup

Butter Beans, most brands (Phases 3 & 4)
13 g Net Carbs per ½ cup

Chickpeas, most brands (Phases 3 & 4)
13 g Net Carbs per ½ cup

Great Northern, most brands (Phases 3 & 4)
14 g Net Carbs per ½ cup

Cannellini, most brands (Phases 3 & 4)
13 g Net Carbs per ½ cup

White Beans, most brands (Phases 3 & 4)
13 g Net Carbs per ½ cup

Black Beans, most brands (Phases 3 & 4)
12 g Net Carbs per ½ cup

USE YOUR BEAN

Make a bean salad using beige or black soybeans. They contain only 4 grams of Net Carbs per ½ cup cooked, compared to 8–15 for most other beans.

CHILIS AND STEWS

FYI **Castleberry's Beef Stew (Phases 3 & 4)**
11 g Net Carbs per cup
  Contains MSG.

Dinty Moore Beef Stew (Phases 3 & 4)
14 g Net Carbs per cup

⚠ Health Valley Mild Vegetarian Chili
19 g Net Carbs per ½ cup
  Contains added sugars.

⚠ **Health Valley Mild Vegetarian Chili with Organic Beans**
19 g Net Carbs per cup
Contains added sugars.

⚠ **Hormel Chili, No Beans**
14 g Net Carbs per cup
Contains added sugars.

⚠ **Hormel Chili with Beans**
26 g Net Carbs per cup
Contains added sugars.

⚠ **Hormel Turkey Chili with Beans**
25 g Net Carbs per cup
Contains added sugars.

SOUPS AND BROTHS

Some canned soups may be low in grams of Net Carbs but still thickened with ingredients like white flour and cornstarch, or loaded with added sugars. Very few canned soups pass muster, so read labels and ingredients lists on individual soups within brands—and visit your natural foods store for more options (see page 360).

⚠ **Campbell's Broccoli Cheese**
14 g Net Carbs per ½ cup
Contains trans fats.

⚠ **Campbell's Cream of Asparagus**
9 g Net Carbs per ½ cup
Contains added sugars.

⚠ **Campbell's Cream of Celery**
9 g Net Carbs per ½ cup
Contains trans fats.

⚠ **Campbell's Cream of Chicken**
10 g Net Carbs per ½ cup
  Contains trans fats.

⚠ **Campbell's Cream of Mushroom**
8 g Net Carbs per ½ cup
  Contains trans fats.

⚠ **Campbell's Oyster Stew**
5 g Net Carbs per ½ cup
  Contains trans fats.

⚠ **Campbell's Tomato**
19 g Net Carbs per ½ cup
  Contains added sugars.

⚠ **Campbell's Chunky Beef Rib Roast**
14 g Net Carbs per cup
  Contains added sugars.

**Campbell's Chunky Hearty Chicken & Vegetables
(Phases 3 & 4)**
11 g Net Carbs per cup

⚠ **Campbell's Healthy Request Chicken Noodle**
7 g Net Carbs per ½ cup
  Contains added sugars.

⚠ **Campbell's Healthy Request Cream of Chicken**
11 g Net Carbs per ½ cup
  Contains trans fats.

⚠ **Campbell's Healthy Request Cream of Mushroom**
8 g Net Carbs per ½ cup
  Contains trans fats.

⚠ **Campbell's Healthy Request Tomato**
17 g Net Carbs per ½ cup
   Contains added sugars.

⚠ **College Inn, Chicken Broth**
0 g Net Carbs per cup
   Contains trans fats and added sugars.

⚠ **College Inn, Beef Broth**
0 g Net Carbs per cup
   Contains trans fats and added sugars.

⚠ **Health Valley Organic, Beef-, Chicken-Flavored Broth**
2 g Net Carbs per cup
   Contains added sugars.

⚠ **Health Valley Organic Black Bean**
20 g Net Carbs per cup
   Contains added sugars.

Imagine Organic No-Chicken Broth (Phases 1-4)
4 g Net Carbs per cup

Imagine Organic Creamy Broccoli (Phases 2-4)
8 g Net Carbs per cup

Imagine Organic Creamy Portobello Mushroom (Phases 2-4)
8 g Net Carbs per cup

Imagine Organic Creamy Potato Leek (Phases 3 & 4)
12 g Net Carbs per cup

Imagine Organic Creamy Sweet Corn (Phases 3 & 4)
4 g Net Carbs per cup

⚠ **Kitchen Basics Stock, Beef, Chicken**
1 g Net Carbs per cup
  Contains added sugars.

Kitchen Basics Stock, Roasted Vegetable (Phases 1-4)
5 g Net Carbs per cup

⚠ **Lipton Cup-a-Soup, Chicken Noodle**
8 g Net Carbs per envelope
  Contains added sugars.

⚠ **Lipton Cup-a-Soup, Vegetable Beef**
6 g Net Carbs per envelope
  Contains trans fats.

Progresso Vegetable Classics, Lentil (Phases 3 & 4)
24 g Net Carbs per cup

⚠ **Progresso Savory Beef Barley Vegetable**
17 g Net Carbs per cup
  Contains added sugars.

⚠ **Progresso Vegetable Classics, Minestrone**
14 g Net Carbs per cup
  Contains added sugars.

FYI **Progresso Homestyle Chicken (Phases 3 & 4)**
10 g Net Carbs per cup
  Contains MSG.

Progresso Steak Beef & Mushroom (Phases 3 & 4)
13 g Net Carbs per cup

⚠ **Rienzi Chicken & Pasta Rotini**
12 g Net Carbs per cup
  Contains added sugars.

⚠ Rienzi Chicken & Rice
15 g Net Carbs per cup
  Contains added sugars.

⚠ Rienzi Minestrone
14 g Net Carbs per cup
  Contains added sugars.

⚠ Swanson 99% Fat Free Chicken Broth
1 g Net Carbs per cup
  Contains added sugars.

FYI Swanson 99% Fat Free Beef Broth (Phases 1-4)
0 g Net Carbs per cup
  Contains MSG.

⚠ Swanson 100% Fat Free Vegetable Broth
3 g Net Carbs per cup
  Contains added sugars.

SOUP'S ON!

Soup is a great appetite controller. Sip a cup of miso soup or reduced-sodium beef, chicken or vegetable broth (add a tablespoon or two of tomato juice for body, if you like) before dinner to fill you up. You won't be tempted to eat as much. Canned cream soups usually have lower carb counts, but beware: They often contain hydrogenated oils.

COCONUT MILK

Take care to buy *unsweetened coconut milk*, not cream of coconut, which comes in a can, too, but is sweetened and much higher in Net Carbs than coconut milk.

Goya (Phases 1-4)
2 g Net Carbs per 2 ounces

A Taste of Thai, unsweetened (Phases 1-4)
2 g Net Carbs per ¼ cup

VEGETABLES

When it comes to canned vegetables and nutrition, there are trade-offs. Exposure to oxygen can decrease the amount of some vitamins in a food; the more time that elapses between the field and your table, the fewer nutrients a vegetable supplies. Large commercial food companies have processing plants by the fields. Foods are harvested and canned within hours, preserving freshness and flavor.

Heat, whether from cooking at your home or the canning process, can also decrease the amount of nutrients, particularly vitamin C, in a food. While you might think that eating fresh, raw vegetables is the answer, heat also helps to break down cell walls in vegetables and increase the availability of other nutrients.

The bottom line? Aim for fresh, local vegetables. When they are not available or you are in a rush, eat a variety of veggies, prepared a variety of ways.

Del Monte Beets (Phases 3 & 4)
6 g Net Carbs per ½ cup

Del Monte Cut Green Beans (Phases 1-4)
2 g Net Carbs per ½ cup

Del Monte Wax Beans (Phases 1-4)
2 g Net Carbs per ½ cup

Del Monte Lima Beans (Phases 3 & 4)
11 g Net Carbs per ½ cup

Del Monte Sliced Carrots (Phases 3 & 4)
5 g Net Carbs per ½ cup

Del Monte Whole Kernel Corn (Phases 3 & 4)
15 g Net Carbs per ½ cup

Del Monte White Corn (Phases 3 & 4)
8 g Net Carbs per ½ cup

Del Monte Fiesta Corn (Phases 3 & 4)
10 g Net Carbs per ½ cup

Del Monte White Corn, Cream Style (Phases 3 & 4)
19 g Net Carbs per ½ cup

Del Monte Peas & Carrots (Phases 3 & 4)
9 g Net Carbs per ½ cup

Del Monte Sweet Peas (Phases 3 & 4)
9 g Net Carbs per ½ cup

Del Monte Zucchini in Tomato Sauce (Phases 1-4)
6 g Net Carbs per ½ cup

Green Giant Cut Asparagus Spears (Phases 1-4)
2 g Net Carbs per 5 spears

Green Giant French Style Green Beans (Phases 1-4)
3 g Net Carbs per ½ cup

Green Giant Cut Green Beans (Phases 1-4)
3 g Net Carbs per ½ cup

Green Giant Three Bean Salad (Phases 3 & 4)
16 g Net Carbs per ½ cup

**Green Giant Whole Kernel Sweet Corn
(Phases 3 & 4)**
15 g Net Carbs per ½ cup

Green Giant Cream Style Sweet Corn (Phases 3 & 4)
18 g Net Carbs per ½ cup

**Green Giant MexiCorn with Red & Green Peppers
(Phases 3 & 4)**
13 g Net Carbs per ⅓ cup

Green Giant Sliced Mushrooms (Phases 1-4)
3 g Net Carbs per can

FRUITS

Choose fruits packed in juice, rather than sugar syrup, even if it is called light syrup, which is unacceptable in any phase of Atkins. Both are higher in grams of Net Carbs than raw fruit, but fruit's own juice doesn't have sugar or sweetener added to it. Drain off the juice to reduce carbs even further. For more information on fruit, see page 53.

⚠ Del Monte Diced Peaches in Extra Light Syrup
12 g Net Carbs per serving
  Contains added sugars.

Del Monte Fresh Cut Sliced Pineapple (Phases 3 & 4)
16 g Net Carbs per serving

Del Monte Fruit Cocktail in 100% Fruit Juice
(Phases 3 & 4)
14 g Net Carbs per ½ cup

Del Monte Orchard Select Sliced Pears
(Phases 3 & 4)
18 g Net Carbs per serving

Del Monte Orchard Select Unpeeled Apricot Halves
(Phases 3 & 4)
20 g Net Carbs per serving

Dole Pineapple Chunks in Pineapple Juice
(Phases 3 & 4)
14 g Net Carbs per ½ cup

Libby's Natural Lite (In Real Fruit Juice), Sliced
Peaches (Phases 3 & 4)
12 g Net Carbs per ½ cup

Libby's 100% Pure Fruit & Juice Bartlett Pear Halves
(Phases 3 & 4)
11 g Net Carbs per ½ cup

Libby's 100% Pure Fruit & Juice Fruit Cocktail
(Phases 3 & 4)
14 g Net Carbs per ½ cup

Libby's 100% Pure Pumpkin (Phases 1-4)
4 g Net Carbs per ½ cup

⚠ **Libby's Easy Pumpkin Pie Mix**
18 g Net Carbs per ½ cup
  Contains added sugars.

Roland Mandarin Oranges in Water (Phases 3 & 4)
9 g Net Carbs per ½ cup

CUT THE CARBS

Some canned fruits are hard to find packed in water. Do not purchase anything in syrup, even light syrup.

BEEF

For more information on beef, see page 89.

Hormel Dried Beef (Phases 1-4)
1 g Net Carbs per 8 slices

⚠ **Libby's Corned Beef**
0 g Net Carbs per 2 ounces
Contains added sugars.

CHICKEN AND TURKEY

For more information on chicken and turkey, see pages 102 and 104 respectively.

Hormel Turkey in Water (Phases 1-4)
0 g Net Carbs per 2 ounces

Swanson Chicken Breast (Phases 1-4)
1 g Net Carbs per 2 ounces

⚠ **Underwood Chicken Spread**
0 g Net Carbs
Contains added sugars and trans fats.

HAM

For more information on ham, see page 92.

Hormel, Ham in Water (Phases 1-4)
0 g Net Carbs per 2 ounces

⚠️ **Hormel Spam, Spam Lite**
1 g Net Carbs per 2 ounces
   Contains added sugars.

⚠️ **Underwood Deviled Ham Spread**
0 g Net Carbs per ¼ cup
   Contains added sugars.

COCKTAIL SAUCE

⚠️ **Crosse & Blackwell**
23 g Net Carbs per 2 tablespoons
   Contains added sugars.

⚠️ **Del Monte**
24 g Net Carbs per 2 tablespoons
   Contains added sugars.

⚠️ **Golden Dipt, Original**
14 g Net Carbs per ¼ cup
   Contains added sugars.

Gold's (Phases 1-4)
2 g Net Carbs per 2 tablespoons

⚠️ **Heinz**
14 g Net Carbs per 2 tablespoons
   Contains added sugars.

⚠️ **Kraft**
12 g Net Carbs per 2 tablespoons
   Contains added sugars.

⚠ Marzetti
0 g Net Carbs per 2 tablespoons
  Contains added sugars.

⚠ Northern Chef
12 g Net Carbs per 2 tablespoons
  Contains added sugars.

⚠ Old Original Bookbinders
14 g Net Carbs per 2 tablespoons
  Contains added sugars.

SEAFOOD

Canned seafood is wonderfully convenient for making delicious low-carb salads—combine canned crab, tuna or shrimp with mayonnaise, herbs and seasonings and chopped celery, and you have a five-minute lunch or light dinner.

Canned tuna comes in three grades: solid or fancy, which is large pieces; smaller-pieced chunk; or bits and pieces, known as flaked. Use tuna packed in oil for heated dishes and water-packed tuna for salads.

Since these foods taste savory, it can be hard to believe that many contain sugar. Be on the lookout for added sugars in the ingredients lists. For more information on fish and seafood, see page 78.

Bumble Bee Crabmeat, Fancy White (Phases 1-4)
0 g Net Carbs per 2 ounces

Bumble Bee Shrimp, Tiny, Medium (Phases 1-4)
0 g Net Carbs per 2 ounces

⚠ Chicken of the Sea Crabmeat, Lump
1 g Net Carbs per ¼ cup
  Contains added sugars.

Mackerel, most brands (Phases 1-4)
2 g Net Carbs per ⅓ cup

Roland Baby Clams (Phases 1-4)
2 g Net Carbs per ½ cup

Roland Smoked Mussels (Phases 1-4)
3 g Net Carbs per ⅓ cup

Roland Smoked Oysters (Phases 1-4)
4 g Net Carbs per ⅓ cup

Salmon, all varieties, most brands (Phases 1-4)
0 g Net Carbs per ¼ cup

Sardines, in oil or water, most brands (Phases 1-4)
0 g Net Carbs per can

Sardines, in tomato sauce, most brands (Phases 2-4)
3 g Net Carbs per can

Snow's Clams, chopped or minced (Phases 1-4)
2 g Net Carbs per ¼ cup

StarKist Premium Tuna Pouch, Albacore, Chunk (Phases 1-4)
0 g Net Carbs per ¼ cup

▲ StarKist Tuna Creations, Sweet & Spicy
3 g Net Carbs per ¼ cup
   Contains added sugars.

Three Diamonds Crabmeat (Phases 1-4)
2 g Net Carbs per 2 ounces

Three Diamonds Smoked Oysters (Phases 1-4)
10 g Net Carbs per can

Tuna, in oil or water, most brands (Phases 1-4)
0 g Net Carbs per 2 ounces

TOMATOES (CANNED)

Pay attention to serving sizes. Yes, you can eat up to one cup of raw tomatoes a day during Induction. However, keep in mind that tomatoes cook down considerably, and you won't be allowed as much of the concentrated forms, like purée and paste. A ½-cup can quickly account for one-quarter of your daily Net Carbs.

Contadina, Crushed with Italian Herbs (Phases 1-4)
3 g Net Carbs per ¼ cup

Contadina, Puree (Phases 1-4)
4 g Net Carbs per ¼ cup

Contadina, Stewed, Italian-Style (Phases 1-4)
7 g Net Carbs per ½ cup

Del Monte Fresh Cut, Diced (Phases 1-4)
4 g Net Carbs per ½ cup

⚠ **Del Monte, Stewed**
7 g Net Carbs per ½ cup
   Contains added sugars.

Muir Glen Organic, Crushed (Phases 1-4)
3 g Net Carbs per ¼ cup

Muir Glen Organic, Diced with Basil & Garlic (Phases 1-4)
3 g Net Carbs per ¼ cup

Muir Glen Organic, Diced, Fire Roasted (Phases 1-4)
5 g Net Carbs per ½ cup

Muir Glen Organic, Ground, Peeled with Basil (Phases 1-4)
2 g Net Carbs per ¼ cup

Muir Glen Organic, Tomato Puree (Phases 1-4)
4 g Net Carbs per ¼ cup

Muir Glen Organic, Whole, Peeled (Phases 1-4)
4 g Net Carbs per ½ cup

Muir Glen Organic, Whole, Peeled with Basil (Phases 2-4)
8 g Net Carbs per ½ cup

Parmalat Pomi Strained Tomatoes (Phases 1-4)
2 g Net Carbs per ½ cup

Progresso, Peeled, Italian Style (Phases 1-4)
3 g Net Carbs per ½ cup

Red Pack, Crushed (Phases 1-4)
4 g Net Carbs per ½ cup

Red Pack, Diced (Phases 1-4)
4 g Net Carbs per ½ cup

Red Pack, Puree (Phases 1-4)
4 g Net Carbs per ¼ cup

Red Pack, Whole, Peeled (Phases 1-4)
4 g Net Carbs per ½ cup

TOMATO AND PASTA SAUCES

Amy's Family Marinara (Phases 2-4)
5 g Net Carbs per ½ cup

Amy's Garlic Mushroom (Phases 2-4)
7 g Net Carbs per ½ cup

⚠ **Amy's Puttanesca**
4 g Net Carbs per ½ cup
    Contains added sugars.

⚠ **Amy's Tomato Basil Sauce**
8 g Net Carbs per ½ cup
    Contains added sugars.

⚠ **Barilla Marinara, Mushroom & Garlic, Roasted Garlic & Onion**
8 g Net Carbs per ½ cup
    Contains added sugars.

⚠ **Bertolli Creamy Alfredo, Original, Garlic, Portobello**
3 g Net Carbs per ¼ cup
    Contains added sugars.

⚠ **Bertolli Tomato & Basil**
7 g Net Carbs per ½ cup
    Contains added sugars.

Carb Options Alfredo Sauce (Phases 1-4)
2 g Net Carbs per ¼ cup

Carb Options Garden Style Sauce (Phases 1-4)
5 g Net Carbs per ½ cup

⚠ **Classico Alfredo, Original, Roasted Garlic**
3 g Net Carbs per ¼ cup
    Contains added sugars.

Classico Florentine Spinach and Cheese (Phases 2-4)
6 g Net Carbs per ½ cup

Classico Four Cheese, Tomato & Basil (Phases 2-4)
7 g Net Carbs per ½ cup

Classico Roasted Peppers & Onion, Spicy Tomato & Pesto, Roasted Garlic (Phases 2-4)
7 g Net Carbs per ½ cup

Classico Spicy Red Pepper (Phases 1-4)
4 g Net Carbs per ½ cup

Classico Tomato Alfredo (Phases 2-4)
5 g Net Carbs per ¼ cup

Colavita Garden Style (Phases 2-4)
9 g Net Carbs per ½ cup

Colavita Marinara (Phases 2-4)
7 g Net Carbs per ½ cup

Colavita Puttanesca (Phases 2-4)
10 g Net Carbs per ½ cup

⚠ Emeril's Kicked Up Tomato
7 g Net Carbs per ½ cup
  Contains added sugars.

⚠ Muir Glen Organic, Garden Vegetable, Italian Herb, Roasted Garlic
10 g Net Carbs per ½ cup
  Contains added sugars.

⚠ Muir Glen Organic Tomato Basil
12 g Net Carbs per ½ cup
  Contains added sugars.

⚠ **Newman's Own Five Cheese, Vodka Sauce, Tomato & Roasted Garlic**
11 g Net Carbs per ½ cup
  Contains added sugars.

Newman's Own Fra Diavolo (Phases 2-4)
7 g Net Carbs per ½ cup

⚠ **Newman's Own Marinara, Mushroom Marinara, Sockarooni**
6 g Net Carbs per ½ cup
  Contains added sugars.

⚠ **Ragu Classic Alfredo**
3 g Net Carbs per ¼ cup
  Contains added sugars.

⚠ **Ragu Flavored with Meat**
5 g Net Carbs per ½ cup
  Contains added sugars.

⚠ **Ragu Marinara**
9 g Net Carbs per ½ cup
  Contains added sugars.

Ragu Rich & Thick Tomato Basil, No Sugar Added (Phases 1-4)
5 g Net Carbs per ¼ cup

Rao's Homemade Marinara, Puttanesca, Arrabiata (Phases 1-4)
5 g Net Carbs per ½ cup

Rao's Homemade Vodka (Phases 1-4)
6 g Net Carbs per ½ cup

Walden Farms No Carb Gourmet Marinara (Phases 1-4)
0 g Net Carbs per ⅓ cup

TOMATO AND PESTO PASTE/SPREADS

Look for pastes and spreads in tubes, rather than cans; Amore is one brand. They are higher priced than the equivalent amount in a can, but you can seal the tubes and store them indefinitely. Once you've opened a can of tomato paste, it can spoil quickly. Paste in tubes is more concentrated than the canned variety, so use half as much. (For anchovy paste and olive paste, see pages 192 and 193 respectively.)

Amore Italian Pesto Paste (Phases 1-4)
3 g Net Carbs per 2 tablespoons

Amore Sun-Dried Tomato Paste (Phases 1-4)
<1 g Net Carbs per teaspoon

Amore Tomato Paste (Phases 1-4)
3 g Net Carbs per 1½ tablespoons

⚠ **Classico Creations Basil Pesto Sauce & Spread**
5 g Net Carbs per ¼ cup
  Contains trans fats.

⚠ **Classico Creations Sun-dried Tomato Pesto Sauce & Spread**
7 g Net Carbs per ¼ cup
  Contains added sugars.

Contadina Tomato Paste (Phases 1-4)
5 g Net Carbs per 2 tablespoons

Hunt's Tomato Paste (Phases 1-4)
4 g Net Carbs per 2 tablespoons

WORST BITES: Pasta sauce can have a huge carb range. Plain and cheese-based sauces tend to be the lowest. But watch out for the occasional exception. Prego Ricotta Garlic Parmesan has 17 grams of Net Carbs per serving and added sugars.

Libby's Easy Pumpkin Pie Mix makes short work of making desserts, but it's a nutritional minefield. Canned pumpkin is sky-high in beta carotene and is a significant source of fiber, vitamins E and C, and iron—for a mere 4 grams of Net Carbs per half-cup. The pie mix, with its sugar and spices, has more than four times the Net Carbs—a whopping 18—per third-cup.

The Pastas, Grains, Beans, and Legumes Aisle

Whole grains, as well as foods made from them, beans and legumes are rich in nutrients, including carbohydrates. During the weight-loss phases of Atkins, these are foods that are mostly absent from your eating plan. However, once you have successfully incorporated seeds and nuts, as well as berries into your menus, you can consider adding back beans; but wait until after you've begun to eat fruits other than berries and starchy vegetables before you add whole grains.

When it comes to pasta, if you thought following a controlled-carb lifestyle meant giving it up forever, you'll be pleased to know that that isn't the case at all. Even in OWL, you can enjoy controlled-carb pasta—delicious tossed with olive oil or butter and sprinkled with freshly grated Parmesan. And in the later phases, depending on your ACE, you can occasionally eat whole-wheat pasta.

➤ GRAINS ◄

WHOLE GRAINS

The final rung on the carbohydrate ladder, whole grains are complex carbohydrates that are digested slowly, and thus have less effect on blood sugar levels than refined grains. They contain varying amounts of protein, B vitamins, and trace minerals.

Barley, pearled (Phases 3 & 4)
19 g Net Carbs per ½ cup cooked

Pearled barley isn't technically a whole grain—the bran has been removed. However, its glycemic index—the impact it has on your blood sugar—is relatively low. Hulled barley contains the germ and most of the bran, but it's rarely available in supermarkets.

Buckwheat Groats (kasha) (Phases 3 & 4)
14 g Net Carbs per ½ cup cooked

Bulgur (Phases 3 & 4)
13 g Net Carbs per ½ cup cooked

Bulgur is a form of whole wheat. The wheat berry is cooked, dried, and then cracked and can either be cooked briefly or soaked in boiling water before eating. When cut fine, it is used for tabouli.

Couscous, whole-wheat (Phases 3 & 4)
17 g Net Carbs per ½ cup cooked

Not a whole grain, couscous is similar to pasta—it's made from semolina dough that has been cut into tiny pieces. On Atkins, whole-wheat couscous is the only form that's acceptable.

Millet (Phases 3 & 4)
19.5 g Net Carbs per ½ cup cooked

A nutritious change of pace from rice, millet is a good source of magnesium and zinc, and supplies thiamin and niacin as well.

Oats (see page 313.)

Rice, brown (Phases 3 & 4)
20.5 g Net Carbs per ½ cup cooked

Brown rice has the bran intact; it has about six times the fiber of white rice. Rice supplies thiamin, niacin, vitamin

B_6, copper, zinc, and magnesium. When you choose rice, keep the portions small.

Rice, white
22 g Net Carbs per ½ cup cooked
Choose brown rice over white, which is highly refined.

Rice, wild (Phases 3 & 4)
16 g Net Carbs per ½ cup cooked
Neither rice nor really wild, this is the seed of an aquatic grass. It's a rich source of folate, zinc, and niacin, and provides almost twice as much protein as does white rice.

GRAIN MIXES

Whole grains are the last rung on the carbohydrate ladder, but they do have a place in your lifetime eating regimen, as long as you keep portions small. Keep in mind that a half-cup portion of grains is about the size of a baseball sliced in half.

Most of the time, grain mixes contain sugar, are very high in sodium or include other unacceptable ingredients, like bleached flour and even potatoes. Fortunately, it's easy to make a seasoned grain-based dish: Sauté a bit of onion and garlic until soft, then add some spices and the grain and sauté until the mixture is wonderfully fragrant and the grains are well coated. Add the liquid and complete cooking; stir in a bit of nuts, or finely chopped red pepper or herbs, just before serving.

⚠ Goya Mexican Rice
37 g Net Carbs per ¼ cup
Contains added sugars.

⚠ Goya Rice and Black Beans
31 g Net Carbs per ¼ cup
Contains added sugars.

Manischewitz Lentil Pilaf (Phases 3 & 4)
29 g Net Carbs per ¼ cup

Manischewitz Rice Pilaf (Phases 3 & 4)
34 g Net Carbs per ¼ cup

Near East Rice Pilaf with Lentils (Phases 3 & 4)
28 g Net Carbs per 1 cup prepared

⚠ Near East Tabouli Wheat Salad
16 g Net Carbs per ⅔ cup prepared
Contains added sugars.

FYI Telma Falafel (Phases 3 & 4)
15 g Net Carbs per 2 tablespoons
Contains wheat flour.

➤ BEANS AND LEGUMES ◄

DRIED BEANS AND LEGUMES

Beans are high in all kinds of vitamins and minerals, as well as fiber, protein, and carbohydrate. Beans also contain antioxidants that can help prevent some types of cancer and protect against heart disease. To cut back on carbs, use them as an "extra," rather than the main ingredient—toss a handful into salads, use in stir-fries or add to soups.

Try to eat beans with vegetables that are high in vitamin C, such as tomatoes. This helps your body absorb the iron from the beans. See page 210 for information on canned beans.

GRAINS EXPLAINED

Grains are voluminously high in carbs. Try these tips when you are ready to incorporate them into your menus:

- Stir a small portion into soup—they can help thicken a meager broth, and they provide flavor and texture.
- Stuff into a pocket cut into a pork chop.
- Toast wheat germ or bran, then sprinkle over yogurt or use as a coating for foods before sautéing.
- To keep portions at the appropriate size, use grains as a component of an entree rather than as a side dish, which can make it all too easy to eat too much.

Like legumes, whole grains are digested slowly, so they are much less likely to wreak havoc on your blood sugar levels than are processed grains such as white rice.

What can you gain from whole grains? As nutrition-rich carbs they are a good source of protein, fiber, vitamin E, several of the B vitamins, and trace minerals such as phosphorus, manganese, zinc and selenium. Just remember to keep your portion size small.

Adzuki (azuki, aduki) (Phases 3 & 4)
20 g Net Carbs per ½ cup cooked
These small, rust-colored beans are fairly high in iron. They are a common ingredient in Japanese cooking.

Black (Phases 3 & 4)
13 g Net Carbs per ½ cup cooked
Sometimes called turtle beans, black beans have a creamy texture and rich flavor.

Black-Eyed Peas (black-eyed beans) (Phases 3 & 4)
12.5 g Net Carbs per ½ cup cooked
These small white beans with black dots provide almost half the daily requirement for folate per serving.

Cannellini (white kidney beans) (Phases 3 & 4)
17 g Net Carbs per ½ cup cooked
Common in Italian cooking, cannellini pair particularly well with bitter greens—add them to sautéed escarole.

Chickpeas (garbanzos) (Phases 3 & 4)
16.5 g Net Carbs per ½ cup cooked
Chickpeas are rich in folate and iron, and in both soluble and insoluble fiber. Take care not to skimp on soaking or cooking these—they're very dense.

Cranberry (Roman) (Phases 3 & 4)
12.5 g Net Carbs per ½ cup cooked
Cranberry beans look like tan kidney beans with cranberry-red speckles; they become tan when cooked.

Fava (broadbean) (Phases 3 & 4)
12 g Net Carbs per ½ cup cooked
Look for fresh favas in the spring. They're a hearty addition to soups.

Great Northern (Phases 3 & 4)
12.5 g Net Carbs per ½ cup cooked
These white beans are fairly high in calcium and have a creamy texture.

Lentils (Phases 3 & 4)
12 g Net Carbs per ½ cup cooked
The most common lentil is the green one—despite its name, it's more of a brownish color—although there are red, yellow, brown and even black ones, which have different

textures when cooked as well. Lentils are an excellent source of folate and iron.

Lima, large (Phases 3 & 4)
13 g Net Carbs per ½ cup cooked

Sometimes called Fordhooks or butterbeans, large limas contain 2.5 grams of sugars. You may find limas in the freezer section as well (see page 291) and for a short season in the produce department.

Lima, baby (Phases 3 & 4)
14 g Net Carbs per ½ cup cooked

Despite their name, baby limas are not simply Fordhooks (see above) that are harvested early—they are a separate, smaller variety.

Navy (Phases 3 & 4)
18 g Net Carbs per ½ cup cooked

Although recipes frequently say that Navy beans and great Northern beans are interchangeable, they're not when you're watching your carbs! Navy beans are considerably higher in Net Carbs than are great Northerns.

Pigeon Peas (Phases 3 & 4)
14 g Net Carbs per ½ cup cooked

Sometimes sold fresh, pigeon peas are about the size of green peas and are almost always split.

Pink (Phases 3 & 4)
19 g Net Carbs per ½ cup cooked

Small and reddish brown, pinks are among the beans with the highest Net Carbs. They're very similar to pinto beans.

Pinto (Phases 3 & 4)
14.5 g Net Carbs per ½ cup cooked
Pink with red stripes when raw, pinto beans look and taste like pink beans when cooked—but with 4.5 fewer grams of Net Carbs per half cup.

Red Kidney (Phases 3 & 4)
14.5 g Net Carbs per ½ cup cooked
Large and dark red, with a firm, almost meaty texture, red kidney beans are often used in chili.

Soybeans (Phases 3 & 4)
6 g Net Carbs per ½ cup cooked
Soybeans are a great source of protein. Look for green soybeans, or edamame, in your grocer's freezer section—boiled and lightly salted, they make a satisfying snack or salad topping.

Split Peas (Phases 3 & 4)
12.5 g Net Carbs per ½ cup cooked
Available in yellow and green, split peas cook quickly and require no soaking.

➤ PASTA ◄

Avoid pasta made from white flour—it has a high-glycemic index, meaning it will elevate your blood sugar *pronto*. Whole-wheat pasta is hardly virtuous, since it is still very high in Net Carbs. And don't be duped by impressive-sounding terms like "semolina" and "durum wheat"—both of these are refined flour made from a very hard wheat specifically suited to making pasta, as opposed to bread or cakes, for example.

Asian noodles aren't always a lower-carb alternative: Rice noodles, somen, and bean threads are actually higher in Net Carbs than regular pasta. Soba noodles, made from buck-

A BETTER WAY WITH BEANS

You know beans are fiber- and nutrient-rich, but you also know
they're high in Net Carbs. When you're ready to add them
back to your meals, use them more sparingly and you'll reap
the benefits without maxing out on carbs. Here are some
ideas:

- Wrap beans, diced tomatoes and a sprinkling of shredded Monterey Jack cheese in an Atkins Bakery Tortilla.
- Scatter beans over a salad; use dark greens like arugula, watercress and romaine, and toss in sliced red bell
  peppers.
- Add ½ cup pureed beans to 1 quart of soup to thicken it
  and give it a rich, creamy texture.
- Make dips, but go beyond hummus, which is made with
  chickpeas. Puree black beans with chili powder and lime
  juice, or puree white beans with sage or rosemary and
  a splash of white wine vinegar. Serve alongside broccoli
  florets, bell pepper strips, blanched cauliflower florets
  and grape tomatoes.
- Stir small cooked beans into fresh salsa for a terrific topping for grilled fish.

wheat, are somewhat lower. Fortunately, controlled-carb
pasta made from soy is now an option (see page 353).

Finally, if you've become used to restaurant-size portions
of pasta, keep in mind that the typical serving at your favorite Italian bistro could be 5 cups—an appropriate portion
is ½ to 1 cup.

Atkins Quick Quisine Pasta Cuts, Penne, Rotini, Spaghetti (Phases 2-4)
5 g Net Carbs per 2 ounces dry

Atkins Quick Quisine Pasta Sides, Fettuccine Alfredo, Pesto Cream (Phases 2-4)
7 g Net Carbs per cup

Atkins Quick Quisine Pasta Sides, Elbows & Cheese (Phases 2-4)
8 g Net Carbs per cup

DeBoles Organic Whole-Wheat Angel Hair, Spaghetti (Phases 3 & 4)
35 g Net Carbs per 2 ounces dry

Hodgson Mill Whole-Wheat Angel Hair, Bow Tie, Penne, Radiatores, Shells, Spaghetti, Spirals (Phases 3 & 4)
28 g Net Carbs per 2 ounces dry

Hodgson Mill Whole-Wheat Spinach Egg Noodles (Phases 3 & 4)
27 g Net Carbs per 2 ounces dry

USE YOUR NOODLE

Controlled-carb pastas give new meaning to the word *mangia!* Indeed, Atkins Quick Quisine Pasta Cuts in any shape, which are made from soy flour and are high in fiber and protein, contain just 5 grams of Net Carbs per serving. Pasta made from semolina (or durum) wheat will set you back a whopping 40 grams of Net Carbs. Most supermarkets now stock controlled-carb pastas; check the labels, though, to be sure they calculate Net Carbs by subtracting the grams of fiber from the total grams of carbohydrates.

The Snacks Aisles

Snacks are far too important to most Americans—and far too important to the bottom line for supermarkets—to be contained in one aisle. Odds are high that savory snacks, like chips, will be in one section (often near beverages) and sweet ones in another. Wherever you find them, most of these snacks are off-limits on Atkins, no matter the phase—and that includes Lifetime Maintenance.

Not only are many snacks sky high in carbs that come from bleached flour and added sugars, hydrogenated oils—read trans fats—also often lurk in snack foods. Fortunately, thanks to a recent FDA ruling requiring trans fats to be listed on Nutrition Facts labels by 2006, many companies will undoubtedly reformulate their foods rather than expose them as the nutrient minefields they are.

Be aware that many so-called "healthful" snacks, such as protein bars, have astronomical carb counts and can contain unacceptable ingredients, such as added sugars.

➤ SWEET SNACKS ◄

APPLESAUCE AND FRUIT PACKS

As long as they're made without additional sugar, fruit packs and applesauce can be added back once you are in Pre-Maintenance. But very few brands don't add juice concentrates or sugar to sweeten them. Most fruits are high in natural sugar (fructose), so sweeteners—high-fructose corn syrup, juice concentrate, or sugar—are unnecessary.

In any case, a piece of fresh fruit with a piece of cheese or some nuts to moderate the impact on your blood sugar might be more satisfying.

Mott's Natural Style Unsweetened Applesauce (Phases 3 & 4)
11g Net Carbs per 4-ounce container

Musselman Lite "No Sugar Added" Applesauce (Phases 3 & 4)
10 g Net Carbs per 4-ounce container

Musselman Lite "No Sugar Added" Fruit 'n Sauce, Raspberry, Strawberry (Phases 3 & 4)
13 g Net Carbs per 4-ounce container

Musselman Lite "No Sugar Added" Fruit 'n Sauce, Peach (Phases 3 & 4)
12 g Net Carbs per 4-ounce container

⚠ **Del Monte Fruit-to-Go, Mandarin Oranges, Diced Peaches**
16 g Net Carbs per 4-ounce container
   Contains added sugars.

⚠ **Del Monte Fruit-to-Go, Mixed Fruit**
17 g Net Carbs per 4-ounce container
   Contains added sugars.

⚠ **Del Monte Lite Fruit & Gel, Peaches in Strawberry Banana Flavored Gel, Mandarin Orange in Orange Gel**
14 g Net Carbs per 4-ounce container
   Contains added sugars.

Dole Fruit Bowls Pineapple Tidbits in Pineapple Juice (Phases 3 & 4)
15 g Net Carbs per 4-ounce container

Dole Fruit Bowls Tropical Fruit (Phases 3 & 4)
14 g Net Carbs per 4-ounce container

⚠ **Dole Fruit Bowls Diced Peaches in Light Syrup**
17 g Net Carbs per 4-ounce container
  Contains added sugars.

SHOP SMART

You'll be a savvy snack shopper if you remember two rules:

1) **There can be tremendous variation within one brand.** For example, Tostitos Natural Corn Chips are made with organic corn, sunflower oil and sea salt. But Tostitos Restaurant-Style Corn Chips contain hydrogenated oils.
2) **Practice label logic.** "Fat-free" doesn't matter when you are doing Atkins, so don't be impressed with Mott's Fat-Free Applesauce and other products labeled as such. "Fat-free" is often a tip-off for added sugars, and that's certainly true in this case: ½ cup of Mott's Fat-Free Applesauce contains a whopping 26 grams of Net Carbs—more than double that of Mott's unsweetened applesauce.

CANDY

These days, many candy manufacturers are rolling out sugar-free or controlled-carb versions of their bestselling confections; they're often mixed in with the other sweets in the candy aisle. If you don't find them there, look to see if they are in the sugar-free section with foods marketed to diabetics. But take heed: Even if they are low in carbs, these candies can still contain added sugars and hydrogenated oils. Plus, it can be difficult to consume just one serving, causing the carbs to add up.

It's also important to note that these products contain sugar alcohols, which at higher levels can cause gastrointestinal symptoms and a laxative effect in some individuals. Be wary of products with more than 15 grams of sugar alcohols per serving.

Atkins Endulge Bits Candies (Phases 2-4)
2 g Net Carbs per ounce

Atkins Endulge Caramel Nut Chew (Phases 2-4)
2 g Net Carbs per bar

Atkins Endulge Chocolate Candy Bars, Chocolate, Chocolate Crunch (Phases 2-4)
2 g Net Carbs per bar

Atkins Endulge Double Milk Chocolate, Double Milk Chocolate Crunch Candy bar (Phases 2-4)
2 g Net Carbs per bar

Atkins Endulge Peanut Butter Cups (Phases 2-4)
2 g Net Carbs per 3-cup package

Atkins Endulge Peanut Caramel Cluster (Phases 2-4)
1 g Net Carb per bar

FYI **Atkins Endulge Wafer Crisp Bars, Mint, Peanut Butter, Chocolate Crème, Vanilla Crème (Phases 2-4)**
4 g Net Carbs per 2-stick pack
    Contains enriched wheat flour.

⚠ Asher's Sugar-Free Caramel Patties
1 g Net Carbs per 2 pieces
    Contains trans fats.

Asher's Sugar-Free Cordial Cherries (Phases 2-4)
3 g Net Carbs per 3 pieces

Asher's Sugar-Free Liquid Caramel Bars (Phases 2-4)
1 g Net Carbs per bar

⚠️ **Fifty-50 Mini Chocolate Bars**
3 g Net Carbs per 8 pieces
  Contains trans fats.

⚠️ **Fifty-50 Peanut Butter Snack Bar**
6 g Net Carbs per 2 bars
  Contains trans fats.

Go Lightly Butterscotch Candies (Phases 2-4)
0 g Net Carbs per 4 pieces

Go Lightly Starlight Mints (Phases 2-4)
0 g Net Carbs per 2 pieces

La Nouba Sugar-Free Imported Belgian Chocolate, most flavors (Phases 2-4)
4 g Net Carbs per bar

⚠️ **Life Savers Crème Savers Sugar-Free Chocolate & Caramel Crème, Strawberry & Crème**
0 g Net Carbs per 5 pieces
  Contains hydrogenated oils and added sugars.

Hershey's Sugar-Free Chocolate Candy (Phases 2-4)
1 g Net Carbs per 5 pieces

Russell Stover Low-Carb French Mint Miniatures (Phases 2-4)
0.2 g Net Carbs per piece

Russell Stover Low-Carb Toffee Squares (Phases 2-4)
0.2 g Net Carbs per 2 pieces

Russell Stover Low-Carb Mint Patties (Phases 2-4)
0.1 g Net Carbs per 2 patties

**Russell Stover Low-Carb Peanut Butter Cups
(Phases 2-4)**
0.8 g Net Carbs per piece

**Russell Stover Low-Carb Peanut Butter Medallions
(Phases 2-4)**
0.7 g Net Carbs per piece

**Russell Stover Low-Carb Milk Chocolate Medallions
(Phases 2-4)**
0.2 g Net Carbs per piece

Russell Stover Low-Carb Pecan Delights (Phases 2-4)
1.1 g Net Carbs per piece

**Sweet'N Low Hard Sugar-Free Candy, all flavors
(Phases 3 & 4)**
0 g Net Carbs per 5 pieces

⚠ **Nestlé Sugar-Free Pecan Turtles**
2 g Net Carbs per 3 pieces
  Contains trans fats.

⚠ **Reese's Sugar-Free Miniature Peanut Butter Cups**
3 g Net Carbs per 5 pieces
  Contains trans fats.

⚠ **Sorbee "Chocolate Lovers," Peanut Butter, Truffles,
Peppermint Patties**
3 g Net Carbs per 5 pieces
  Contains trans fats.

Sorbee Crystal Light Hard Candy, Assorted Fruit, Lemonade (Phases 2-4)
0 g Net Carbs per 4 pieces

Sorbee Lites Hard Candy, Butterscotch, Assorted Chocolate, Coffee, Fruit (Phases 2-4)
0 g Net Carbs per 4 pieces

Sorbee Sugar-Free Starlite Mints, Lollypops (Phases 2-4)
0 g Net Carbs per 3 pieces

⚠ **Sorbee Sugar-Free Creamy Caramels**
0 g Net Carbs per 7 pieces
   Contains trans fats.

⚠ **Sorbee Sugar-Free Fruit Chews**
0 g Net Carbs per 6 pieces
   Contains trans fats.

Sorbee Sugar-Free Gummy Bears (Phases 2-4)
0 g Net Carbs per 16 pieces

FYI **Sorbee Sugar-Free Frugeli, Jelly Candy (Phases 2-4)**
0 g Net Carbs per 4 pieces
   Contains aspartame.

Sorbee Zero Sugar Fine European Chocolate, Milk, Dark, Milk with Peanuts (Phases 2-4)
0-1 g Net Carbs per ½ bar

Think Thin Low Carb Candy, Chocolate Peanuts, Chocolate Almonds, Chocolate T&T's, Gummy Bears, Sour Worms, Jelly Beans, Sour Citrus Slices, Gum Drops (Phases 2-4)
0-10 g Net Carbs per serving, varies by item

CANDY CAN BE DANDY . . . WITH CAUTION

Controlled-carb candy. It seems like a dream come true—and it can be, if you enjoy it in moderation. When you are primarily burning fat for energy in the early phases of Atkins, there is a natural appetite-controlling mechanism. By the end of OWL (when you are able to have many controlled-carb sweets) and certainly by the time you've reached Lifetime Maintenance, however, you'll have to rely more on self-control.

While you can indulge in the occasional treat, such foods can be hard to eat in small quantities. And just because it is controlled-carb, that doesn't mean you can eat more. Set out the appropriate portion and be firm with yourself about not going back for more. If you find that you are incapable of practicing moderation, it may be easier to stay away from these things altogether and satisfy your sweet tooth with berries and whipped cream.

PROTEIN AND NUTRITION BARS

The protein and nutrition bar rack can be one of the most head-spinning areas of the supermarket. It seems every company, with every nutritional philosophy, has a line of bars in a never-ending list of flavors and textures, not to mention those that contain mysterious-sounding ingredients, fortification and added nutrients.

With so many bars on the market, there are too many to mention here, so we've collected a sampling, in various flavors, that we saw on the shelves in supermarkets. We've also listed a few with exorbitant amounts of Net Carbs for comparison. When evaluating bars, look for carb counts of no more than 3 grams of Net Carbs per bar—and make sure there are no added sugars or hydrogenated oils. Keep in mind, too, a bar that is dubbed "high-protein" is not necessarily low in carbs.

Atkins Advantage Bars, Chocolate Peanut Butter, Almond Brownie, Chocolate Coconut, Cookies 'n Crème, Chocolate Decadence (Phases 1-4)
2 g Net Carbs per bar

Atkins Advantage Bars, S'mores, Chocolate Mocha Crunch (Phases 1-4)
3 g Net Carbs per bar

⚠ **Balance Bars Original, most flavors**
21 g Net Carbs per bar
   Contains added sugars.

Biochem Strive Low Carb Bars, Dark Chocolate Raspberry Crunch (Phases 2-4)
3 g Net Carbs per bar

⚠ **Carb Options, Chocolate Chip Brownie, Chocolate Peanut Butter, Cinnamon Delight**
2 g Net Carbs per bar
   Contains trans fats.

⚠ **Carborite Crispy Nutrition Bars, most flavors**
1-2 g Net Carbs per bar
   Contains added sugars.

CarbSense Aramana Soy Energy Bars, Blueberry Crisp, Mocha Cappuccino Crisp (Phases 2-4)
4 g Net Carbs per bar

CarbSense Aramana Soy Energy Bar, Peanut Butter Crisp (Phases 1-4)
3 g Net Carbs per bar

CarbSense Aramana Soy Energy Bar, Chocolate Crisp (Phases 1-4)
2 g Net Carbs per bar

Carb Solutions High Protein Bar, Chocolate Fudge Almond (Phases 1-4)
3 g Net Carbs per bar

Carb Wise Protein Bar, Lemon Yogurt (Phases 2-4)
4 g Net Carbs per bar

Carb Wise Protein Bar, Chocolate Raspberry (Phases 1-4)
3 g Net Carbs per bar

Carb Wise Protein Bar, Chocolate Peanut Crunch (Phases 1-4)
3 g Net Carbs per bar

Doctor's CarbRite Diet Bars, most flavors (Phases 1-4)
2 g Net Carbs per bar

EAS Myoplex CarbSense Nutrition Bars, Lemon Cheesecake, Apple Cinnamon (Phases 1-4)
3 g Net Carbs per bar

EAS Myoplex CarbSense Nutrition Bar, Cookies & Cream (Phases 1-4)
2 g Net Carbs per bar

⚠️ **EAS Myoplex Storm, Chocolate Peanut Caramel**
29 g Net Carbs per bar
  Contains added sugars.

GeniSoy Low Carb Crunch Bar, Chocolate, Chocolate Chip, Lemon, Peanut Butter, Raspberry
(Phases 1-4)
2 g Net Carbs per bar

Glenny's Slim Carb Big Crunch Bars, Brownie Cheesecake, Double Fudge, Peanut Caramel
(Phases 1-4)
2 g Net Carbs per bar

Keto Blueberry Cheesecake, Caramel Nut Crunch, Chocolate Peanut Butter Cup, Lemon Chiffon
(Phases 1-4)
2 g Net Carbs per bar

Keto Chocolate Coconut Crème, Oatmeal Raisin Crunch and Chocolate Fudge (Phases 1-4)
3 g Net Carbs per bar

Keto Cookies 'n Crème, Chocolate Fudge
(Phases 2-4)
4 g Net Carbs per bar

Lo Carb Deluxe Zero Sugar Protein Bars, most flavors
(Phases 2-4)
2 g Net Carbs per bar

Luna Bar Low-Carb Glow, Chocolate Peanut Crunch, Fudge Almond Brownie, Strawberry Caramel Sundae
(Phases 1-4)
3 g Net Carbs per bar

⚠ **NuGo Peanut Butter Pleaser Bar**
25 g Net Carbs per bar
  Contains added sugars.

⚠️ **Power Bar, Vanilla Crisp, Chocolate Peanut Butter**
42 g Net Carbs per bar
  Contains added sugars.

⚠️ **Power Bar, French Vanilla Crisp**
16 g Net Carbs per bar
  Contains added sugars.

Premier Nutrition Odyssey Triple Layer Protein Bar, Caramel Nut (Phases 2-4)
4 g Net Carbs per bar

Slim-Fast Succeed Low Carb Snack Bars, Chocolate Peanut Butter, Cookies 'n Cream, Banana Nut (Phases 1-4)
2-3 g Net Carbs per bar, varies by flavor

⚠️ **Slim-Fast Low Carb Meal Bars, Chocolate Peanut Butter, Chocolate Brownie, Cinnamon Bun**
2 g Net Carbs per bar
  Contains trans fats.

⚠️ **Tiger's Milk Protein Bar**
17 g Net Carbs per bar
  Contains added sugars.

Think Thin Low Carb Nutrition Bars, Chocolate, French Toast, Caramel, Chunky Peanut, Creamy Peanut Butter, Lemon Meringue, Mixed Berry (Phases 1-4)
2 g Net Carbs per bar

⚠️ **Think Thin Low Carb Nutrition Bar, S'mores**
2 g Net Carbs per bar
  Contains added sugars.

> 🚫 **WORST BITES:** Nutrition bars might be chock-full of vitamins and protein, but they can also be carbohydrate mine fields: Met Rx Big 100 Meal Replacement Bars win the booby prize with 49–53 grams of Net Carbs per bar. Kashi Go Lean Bars are first runner up—the various flavors contain between 42–44 grams of Net Carbs per bar.

GELATIN MIXES

Sugar-free gelatin is acceptable even during Induction, but don't add any berries until you reach OWL, or other fruit until you reach Pre-Maintenance. But feel free to add a dollop of whipped cream, sweetened with Splenda, if you wish.

Hunt's Splenda-Sweetened Juicy Gells, Strawberry, Orange (Phases 1-4)
1 g Net Carbs per serving

Jolly Rancher Sugar-Free Raspberry Gel (Phases 1-4)
2 g Net Carbs per serving

FYI Jell-O Sugar-Free, all flavors (Phases 2-4)
0 g Net Carbs per ½ cup dry
  Contains aspartame.

⚠ Jell-O, regular, all flavors
19 g Net Carbs per ½ cup dry
  Contains added sugars.

PUDDING MIXES

If you like puddings, look for recipes to make them from scratch. It's very easy, and you'll be able to use sucralose instead of aspartame or sugar in your version.

⚠ **Jell-O Pudding & Pie Filling Cook & Serve Vanilla, Chocolate**
20 g Net Carbs per ¼ package
  Contains added sugars.

⚠ **Jell-O Pudding & Pie Filling Cook & Serve Sugar-Free Vanilla, Chocolate**
56 g Net Carbs per ¼ package
  Contains trans fats.

FYI **Jell-O Pudding & Pie Filling Instant Sugar-Free, Fat-Free Vanilla, Chocolate (Phases 2-4)**
6-7 g Net Carbs per ¼ package
  Contains aspartame.

➤ SAVORY SNACKS ◄

Crunchy, salty snacks can pack a double wallop: They're typically high in carbs and made with bleached flour, and they are almost *always* made with hydrogenated oils, meaning they are high in trans fats. The government recently ruled that foods must have trans fats listed on Nutrition Facts labels by 2006. Some companies have begun to change their formulations, so you should check labels to see if your favorite controlled-carb snack is now being made without them.

Your best snack bets are those foods that are minimally processed. Nuts and popcorn are smarter choices than cheese puffs with that nuclear orange glow or vegetable snacks that look more like Styrofoam than anything that came from the earth.

CORN CHIPS

Don't be fooled by "natural" chips: They may contain fewer additives, but they're about the same in grams of Net

Carbs. If you don't have a scale to weigh out an ounce, look to see if the number of chips is listed in the serving size. If it is, count out the number of pieces—or count out half the number of chips for half the grams of Net Carbs.

Bearitos Cheddar Puffs (Phases 3 & 4)
16 g Net Carbs per 2 cups

Bearitos Tortilla Chips, Organic Yellow Corn, White Corn (Phases 3 & 4)
17 g Net Carbs per 15 chips

Bearitos Tortilla Chips, Stone Ground Blue (Phases 3 & 4)
16 g Net Carbs per 15 chips

⚠ Bugles, most flavors
18 g Net Carbs per 1⅓ cup
   Contains trans fats.

FYI Chex Mix (Phases 3 & 4)
18 g Net Carbs per ½ cup
   Contains wheat flour.

⚠ Doritos Edge
6 g Net Carbs per serving
   Contains added sugars.

Frito's, Original (Phases 3 & 4)
18 g Net Carbs per 32 chips

GeniSoy Low Carb Tortilla Chips, Fiesta Salsa, Lightly Salted, Nacho Cheese, Zesty Habanero (Phases 2-4)
8 g Net Carbs per 15 chips

Garden of Eatin' Blue Corn Tortilla Chips (Phases 3 & 4)
16 g Net Carbs per 15 chips

Garden of Eatin' Little Soy Blues Tortilla Chips (Phases 3 & 4)
15 g Net Carbs per 13 chips

Garden of Eatin' White Corn Tortilla Chips (Phases 3 & 4)
17 g Net Carbs per 10 chips

Garden of Eatin' Chili & Lime Tortilla Chips (Phases 3 & 4)
16 g Net Carbs per 10 chips

Garden of Eatin' Red Corn Tortilla Chips (Phases 3 & 4)
17 g Net Carbs per 15 chips

Robert's American Gourmet, The Dude's Chips (Phases 3 & 4)
15 g Net Carbs per ounce

Tostitos, Natural Blue, Natural Yellow (Phases 3 & 4)
18 g Net Carbs per 7 chips

⚠ **Tostitos Edge**
6 g Net Carbs per serving
  Contains added sugars.

POPCORN

Popcorn increases in volume dramatically when cooked: One half-cup unpopped kernels can yield more than 10 cups when popped. Flavored varieties often include modified food starches and other ingredients that inflate the carb count, so stick with the plain stuff.

Bearitos Lite Butter Flavor Popcorn (Phases 3 & 4)
18 g Net Carbs per 3½ cups popped

FALSE FRIENDS:
UNEXPECTED CARBS & TRANS-FAT ALERT

If you spend a lot of time cruising the snack aisles or reading the advertising circulars that come in the Sunday newspapers, you may have seen "healthy" snacks—they're often touted as being much more nutritious (or at least less harmful!) than the regular versions. Don't be fooled. If something sounds too good to be true, it probably is.

- **Baked chips:** These are lower in fat than regular fried potato and corn chips, but weigh in with significantly higher Net Carb counts of 22 grams per serving (on average). In addition, many are loaded with sugar and hydrogenated oils.
- **Mini rice cakes:** On average, these possess a moderate Net Carb count of 12 grams per serving. Although most are designed to be healthy, many contain refined white rice and corn—there are also good and bad choices within the same brand. Some Quaker Mini Rice Cakes are acceptable in the later phases of the ANA, but Quaker's Creamy Ranch Mini Rice Cakes are made with partially hydrogenated oils.
- **Peanut butters:** With an average of 5 grams of Net Carbs per serving, peanut butter seems like a good deal. Take a look at the labels of major brands. Skippy, Jif and Peter Pan all contain hydrogenated oils, and some are sweetened with high-fructose corn syrup.

Bearitos White Cheddar Popcorn (Phases 3 & 4)
14 g Net Carbs per 2⅓ cups popped

⚠ **Newman's Own Microwave, Natural, Butter**
13 g Net Carbs per 3½ cups popped
   Contains trans fats.

⚠ **Orville Redenbacher Butter Popcorn**
13 g Net Carbs per 2 tablespoons unpopped
   Contains trans fats.

Smart Food White Cheddar (Phases 3 & 4)
13 g Net Carbs per cup popped

PORK RINDS AND CRACKLINGS

   The ingredients for these zero-carb items are basic: pork skins and salt. Avoid flavored or sweetened versions.

Most brands
0 g Net Carbs per serving

POTATO CHIPS

   The best-tasting potato chips rarely have more than three ingredients: potatoes, vegetable oil and salt. If the bag you've picked up has more than that, put it back and continue your search—odds are high that buried in the ingredients list are terms like "partially hydrogenated oils" and "modified food starch," neither of which you want or need. (Regional or boutique brands like Cape Cod are more likely to limit the number of ingredients.)
   As you can imagine, this is one food you'll want to eat rarely and in very small quantities and only in the Lifetime Maintenance and Pre-Maintenance phases of Atkins. Servings are usually given in ounces—there are approximately 19 chips in an ounce.

Cape Cod Classic (Phases 3 & 4)
15 g Net Carbs per ounce

Good Health Olive Oil Potato Chips, Cracked Pepper (Phases 3 & 4)
16 g Net Carbs per ounce

Kettle Chips Lightly Salted (Phases 3 & 4)
14 g Net Carbs per ounce

Terra Exotic Potato (Phases 3 & 4)
13 g Net Carbs per ounce

Terra Original (Phases 3 & 4)
15 g Net Carbs per ounce

Terra Sweet Potato Frites (Phases 3 & 4)
13 g Net Carbs per ounce

⚠ **Terra Frites Americaine**
15 g Net Carbs per ounce
  Contains added sugars.

SOY AND VEGETABLE CHIPS

Soy- and vegetable-based chips can be a great alternative to traditional salty snacks. However, not all are low in carbs or free of unacceptable ingredients.

Atkins Crunchers Chips, Original, BBQ (Phases 2-4)
4 g Net Carbs per 1-ounce bag

Atkins Crunchers Chips, Sour Cream and Onion, Nacho (Phases 2-4)
5 g Net Carbs per 1-ounce bag

CarbSense Soy Tortilla Chips, Original, Nacho Cheese, Habanero, Pico de Gallo (Phases 2-4)
8 g Net Carbs per 15 chips

GeniSoy Deep Sea Salted Soy (Phases 3 & 4)
12 g Net Carbs per 25 chips

GeniSoy Creamy Ranch Soy (Phases 3 & 4)
13 g Net Carbs per ounce

GeniSoy Apple Cinnamon Crunch Soy (Phases 3 & 4)
15 Net Carbs per ounce

**Robert's American Gourmet Veggie Chips
(Phases 3 & 4)**
18 g Net Carbs per ounce

**Robert's American Gourmet Girlfriend Booty
(Phases 2-4)**
5 g Net Carbs per ounce

Terra Vegetable Spiced Taro (Phases 3 & 4)
16 g Net Carbs per ounce

PUFFED SNACKS

Look for other lower-carb cheese-flavored snacks, like Just The Cheese bars and rounds, in the natural foods store. Each serving has just 1 gram of Net Carbs.

**Cheeto's Natural White Cheddar Cheese Puffs
(Phases 3 & 4)**
15 g Net Carbs per ounce

**Robert's American Gourmet Smart Puffs
(Phases 3 & 4)**
15 g Net Carbs per ounce

**Robert's American Gourmet Veggie Booty
(Phases 3 & 4)**
17 g Net Carbs per ounce

DON'T GET BENT OUT OF SHAPE

What's a snack food that can really twist your eating the wrong way? Pretzels. Often touted as a healthful snack, they are actually made with white flour and are dense with carbs. Compare pretzels to the other famous betcha-can't-eat-just-one snack, potato chips:

- 10 potato chips = 9.7 grams Net Carbs
- 10 small pretzel twists = 23 grams Net Carbs

For lower-carb alternatives made from soy flour, see pages 319–323.

RICE AND CORN CAKES

While these once had a reputation as "diet food," if you've looked on a package lately, you know that these lighter-than-air snacks are hardly low in carbs. You'll also want to check the ingredients labels carefully, avoiding those that are made with white rice, which is highly refined, and caramel and other sweet-flavored versions, which are filled with molasses and other added sugars.

Hain Mini Munchies, Plain (Phases 3 & 4)
13 g Net Carbs per 14 cakes

Lundberg Brown Rice Cakes (Phases 3 & 4)
15 g Net Carbs per cake

**Quaker Rice Cakes, Plain, Lightly Salted
(Phases 3 & 4)**
7 g Net Carbs per cake

**Quaker Corn Cakes, Butter, White Cheddar
(Phases 3 & 4)**
7 g Net Carbs per cake

⚠ Hain Mini Munchies, Apple Cinnamon, Honey Nut
13-14 g Net Carbs per 9 cakes
  Contains added sugars.

⚠ Hain Mini Munchies, Peanut Butter
12 g Net Carbs per 9 cakes
  Contains added sugars.

⚠ Hain Mini Munchies, Ranch
9 g Net Carbs per 9 cakes
  Contains added sugars.

⚠ Quaker Rice Cakes, Apple Cinnamon
11 g Net Carbs per cake
  Contains added sugars.

NUTS AND SEEDS

Nuts and seeds are among the first foods you add back to your eating plan as you climb the carbohydrate ladder. In addition to being relatively low in carbs, they are also rich sources of protein, beneficial fats, fiber and a wide array of other nutrients: Almonds are a good source of calcium, walnuts are high in omega-3 fats, pecans in thiamin, hazelnuts in vitamin E.

There's very little difference in carbs between dry-roasted and oil-roasted nuts, but skip the honey-roasted or seasoned varieties. Nuts are also pretty consistent in Net Carbs from one brand to another.

The most accurate way to measure a serving of nuts is to weigh it. If you have a food scale, by all means use it to measure out a 1-ounce portion. If you don't, use the serving information that follows to calculate 1 ounce. While we have included soy nuts here, they are actually not "nuts"—they're made by roasting whole, water-soaked dried soybeans.

Almonds, roasted, salted (Phases 2-4)
2 g Net Carbs per ¼ cup (about 25 nuts)

Brazil Nuts (Phases 2-4)
2 g Net Carbs per ¼ cup (6-8 nuts)

Cashews (Phases 2-4)
8 g Net Carbs per ¼ cup (about 18 nuts)

Hazelnuts (Phases 2-4)
1 g Net Carbs per ¼ cup (about 25 nuts)

Macadamia Nuts, roasted, salted (Phases 2-4)
1 g Net Carbs per ¼ cup (10-12 nuts)

Mixed Nuts (Phases 2-4)
4-6 g Net Carbs per ¼ cup (about 35 nuts)

Peanuts, cocktail (Phases 2-4)
4 g Net Carbs per ¼ cup (about 45 nuts)

Peanuts, dry-roasted (Phases 2-4)
3 g Net Carbs per ¼ cup (about 45 nuts)

Pecans (Phases 2-4)
3 g Net Carbs per ¼ cup (about 20 halves)

Pinenuts (Phases 2-4)
3-5 g Net Carbs per ¼ cup (about 2 handfuls)

Pistachios, dry-roasted, salted in shell (Phases 2-4)
6 g Net Carbs per ¼ cup (about 45 nuts)

Pumpkin Seeds (pepitas) (Phases 2-4)
4 g Net Carbs per ¼ cup (about 2 handfuls)

Soybean "Nuts" (Phases 2-4)
6 g Net Carbs per ¼ cup (about 2 handfuls)

Sunflower Seeds, roasted, salted (Phases 2-4)
2 g Net Carbs per ¼ cup (about 2 handfuls)

Walnuts (Phases 2-4)
3 g Net Carbs per ¼ cup (about 14 halves)

NUTS FOR NUTS?

If you aren't one to nosh on nuts, you should be. They are high in protein, fiber, flavor, and healthy fat, and fairly low in carbohydrates. Macadamias and hazelnuts are the lowest in carbs, but almonds, Brazil nuts, and walnuts are runners up.

Nuts do contain some carbs, though, so you should limit your portions to 1 ounce, or about one-quarter cup. To learn what a serving size looks like, measure that amount into the palm of your hand. That way, the next time you are helping yourself to a bowl of nuts at a party, you'll know your limit. (If you find it too difficult to stop eating nuts, buy only individual-size portions.)

What nut is off limits? Anything honey-roasted. The sugar boosts the carb count and undermines the nutritional value.

➤ OTHER SNACKS ◄

PEANUT BUTTERS

When it comes to peanut (and other nut) butters, natural is better. Many major brands contain hydrogenated oils and are loaded with high-fructose corn syrup and other sweeteners. The freshest, most wholesome peanut butter is the kind ground right in your supermarket or health food store. Be sure to keep it in the refrigerator so it doesn't become rancid. For other nut and seed butters, see page 351.

Arrowhead Mills 100% Valencia Creamy Peanut Butter (Phases 2-4)
5 g Net Carbs per 2 tablespoons

⚠ **Carb Options Creamy Peanut Butter**
3 g Net Carbs per 2 tablespoons
 Contains trans fats.

⚠ **Fifty-50 No Added Sugar Peanut Butter**
4 g Net Carbs per 2 tablespoons
 Contains trans fats.

⚠ **Jif Creamy Peanut Butter**
5 g Net Carbs per 2 tablespoons
 Contains trans fats.

**Maple Grove Farms All Natural Creamy Peanut Butter
(Phases 2-4)**
4 g Net Carbs per 2 tablespoons

⚠ **Peter Pan Creamy Peanut Butter**
4 g Net Carbs per 2 tablespoons
 Contains trans fats.

⚠ **Skippy Creamy Peanut Butter**
5 g Net Carbs per 2 tablespoons
 Contains trans fats.

Smucker's Creamy Natural Peanut Butter (Phases 2-4)
5 g Net Carbs per 2 tablespoons

PUMPIN' PROTEIN

Avoid the snack-addiction trap: Rather than reach for carb-based nibbles, opt for a high-protein or high-fat nosh instead. You'll feel satisfied more rapidly.

JERKY

Jerky might seem like a perfect controlled-carb snack—it's made from beef, after all—but that's an erroneous assumption. Once upon a time, jerky was indeed beef that had been dried, and sometimes salted or seasoned. Today, it's often cured with nitrates, and the seasons in the curing mixture often contain sugars. Read the ingredients lists carefully on these products.

⚠ **Oberto Natural-Style Beef**
7 g Net Carbs per ounce
   Contains added sugars.

⚠ **Pemmican Hickory-Smoked Beef**
3 g Net Carbs per ounce
   Contains added sugars.

⚠ **Slim Jim Beef Jerky**
1 g Net Carbs per ounce
   Contains added sugars.

CHEESE SPREADS

⚠ **Kraft Cheez Whiz**
4 g Net Carbs per 2 tablespoons
   Contains added sugars.

FYI **Kraft Easy Cheese (Phases 1-4)**
2 g Net Carbs per 2 tablespoons
   Contains MSG.

The Beverage Aisle

➤ NONALCOHOLIC DRINKS ◄

This is the best of aisles, this is the worst of aisles. Beverages can be your greatest ally or your downfall when it comes to losing and controlling weight. Liquids can help to fill you up, and if your quaff is non-caloric, you won't add Net Carbs. Sugary sodas, sports drinks, sweetened elixirs and teas are all to be avoided, and you'll do yourself a favor if you limit your consumption of caffeinated drinks, which are actually dehydrating and can impact blood sugar when consumed in excess.

Water, of course, is crucial, and as part of the Atkins Nutritional Approach™, you should get at least eight 8-ounce glasses per day. Water is vital for proper cell function and it helps to prevent constipation. Because you've probably upped your fiber intake since you began doing Atkins, getting those glasses is even more critical. You can choose plain, mineral, or spring water. For additional fluids, you can also have seltzer, but do note that the bubbles can fill you up and prevent you from getting all eight glasses. Try one of the new flavor-infused still waters, if you like—they're terrific for satisfying a juice craving—do make sure it's unsweetened or sweetened with sucralose (Splenda).

Hot drinks can curb your appetite. Studies have shown that people who begin a meal with soup eat less, so try a hot broth, or have a cup of unsweetened herbal tea as you prepare dinner. And remember to add in the beverages you consume to your daily Net Carb gram tally—they count, too.

HOT DRINKS

Because many hot drinks contain milk, they're not allowed during Induction. If you're craving something warming, make your own hot drink with decaf coffee or tea, or unsweetened cocoa, cream and sucralose.

Decaf Coffee (Phases 1-4)
0 g Net Carbs per cup

Decaf Black Tea (Phases 1-4)
0 g Net Carbs per cup

Herbal Tea (Phases 1-4)
0 g Net Carbs per cup

Unsweetened Cocoa (Phases 1-4)
1 g Net Carbs per 2 tablespoons

⚠ **General Foods International Coffees Original, all flavors**
10 g Net Carbs per 1⅓ tablespoons
  Contains trans fats and added sugars.

⚠ **General Foods International Coffees, Sugar-Free, all flavors**
5 g Net Carbs per 1⅓ tablespoons
  Contains trans fats.

Swiss Miss Diet Hot Cocoa Mix (Phases 1-4)
3 g Net Carbs per envelope

BEWARE THE WARMING CUP

Ah . . . that sugar-free cup of hot cocoa. Yes, the carb counts are relatively low, but many brands are sweetened with aspartame, and they often contain hydrogenated oils. Look for varieties made with sucralose. A bonus: These are often made without partially hydrogenated oils. If you're having trouble finding one that is acceptable, visit your natural foods store where you'll find controlled-carb brands like McSteven's and Keto.

ICED TEA AND LEMONADE

Atkins Green Tea Blend (Phases 1-4)
0 g Net Carbs per 8 ounces

Arizona No-Carb Green Teas, both flavors (Phases 1-4)
0 g Net Carbs per 8 ounces

Arizona Diet Green Tea (Phases 1-4)
1 g Net Carbs per 8 ounces

Arizona Diet Black Teas, all flavors (Phases 1-4)
0 g Net Carbs per 8 ounces

⚠️ **Arizona Total Trim, most flavors**
1-2 g Net Carbs per 8 ounces
   Contains added sugars.

Carb Options Lemon Flavored Iced Tea Mix (Phases 1-4)
0 g Net Carbs per 8 ounces prepared

FYI **Crystal Light, all flavors (Phases 1-4)**
0 g Net Carbs per 8 ounces
　Contains aspartame.

Diet Snapple Tea, Lime Green, Peach, Raspberry (Phases 1-4)
1 g Net Carbs per 8 ounces

⚠️ **Diet Snapple Apple**
4 g Net Carbs per 8 ounces
　Contains added sugars.

4C Light Iced Tea Mix, all flavors (Phases 1-4)
4 g Net Carbs per 8 ounces

FYI **Kool-Aid Unsweetened Mix (Phases 2-4)**
0 g Net Carbs per 8 ounces
　Contains aspartame.

FYI **Lipton Light Iced Tea Mix, all flavors (Phases 1-4)**
1 g Net Carbs per tablespoon
　Contains aspartame.

Nantucket Nectars Diet Lemon Tea (Phases 1-4)
1 g Net Carbs per 8 ounces

JUICE

　Nearly all bottled juices contain added sugars. Whole fruit is a better choice over fruit juice when it comes to saving on carbs. But if you must have juice, fresh squeezed, pure 100% juice is the best option. (See page 129 for information about juices available in the dairy section.)

Ocean Spray Light, all flavors (Phases 3 & 4)
10 g Net Carbs per cup

Ocean Spray 100% Grapefruit Juice (Phases 3 & 4)
24 g Net Carbs per cup

V-8 Diet Splash, all flavors (Phases 2-4)
3 g Net Carbs per cup

Sacramento Tomato Juice (Phases 2-4)
8 g Net Carbs per cup

⚠️ **Mott's Clamato Tomato Juice Cocktail**
11 g Net Carbs per cup
  Contains added sugars.

MILK AND SOYMILK
(IN ASCEPTIC PACKAGES AND DRY)

Did you know that most soymilk, even plain, is sweet-ened? You won't find sugar or high-fructose corn syrup on the label, but barley syrup, rice syrup and cane juice are often added. Choose soymilk that is unsweetened and do a little research among brands, since some are lower in carbs than others. (See pages 125 and 349 for more information on soymilk.)

Alba Nonfat Dry Milk (Phases 3 & 4)
11 g Net Carbs per 1 cup prepared

⚠️ **Edensoy Original Soymilk**
12 g Net Carbs per cup
  Contains added sugars.

Edensoy Unsweetened Organic Soymilk (Phases 2-4)
3 g Net Carbs per cup

Nestlé Carnation Nonfat Dry Milk (Phases 3 & 4)
12 g Net Carbs per 1 cup prepared

Parmalat Whole, 1%, and Fat-Free Milk (Phases 3 & 4)
12 g Net Carbs per cup

WestSoy Slender, Vanilla, Chocolate, Cappuccino (Phases 1-4)
1 g Net Carbs per cup

WestSoy Unsweetened, Chocolate, Vanilla (Phases 1-4)
2 g Net Carbs per cup

WestSoy Unsweetened, Plain (Phases 1-4)
1 g Net Carbs per cup

White Wave Silk Unsweetened Organic Soymilk (Phases 2-4)
4 g Net Carbs per cup

FALSE FRIENDS: SWEETENED SOY DRINKS

Soymilk is a healthful alternative to dairy, but make sure you seek out unsweetened soy drinks. Some sweetened soymilks have more than nine times the grams of Net Carbs of unsweetened versions! Just take a look at the difference:
- Edensoy Unsweetened Organic *3 g Net Carbs per cup*
- Edensoy Original *12 g Net Carbs per cup*
- Edensoy Vanilla *24 g Net Carbs per cup*
- Edensoy Carob *27 g Net Carbs per cup*

READY-TO-DRINK SHAKES AND DRINK MIXES

Be leery of shakes that tout themselves as being acceptable for diabetics—most of these contain sugar!

Atkins Advantage Ready-to-Drink Shakes, Creamy Vanilla, Chocolate Delight (Phases 1-4)
1 g Net Carbs per can

Atkins Advantage Ready-to-Drink Shakes, Chocolate Royale, Café au Lait, Strawberry Supreme (Phases 1-4)
2 g Net Carbs per can

Atkins Advantage Shake Mixes, all flavors (Phases 1-4)
3 g Net Carbs per 2-scoop serving

Atkins Morning Start Drink Mixes, Orange, Peach Tea, Apple and Fruit Punch (Phases 1-4)
0 g Net Carbs per 8 ounces

⚠ **Alba's Vanilla Dairy Shake Mix**
10 g Net Carbs per packet
  Contains trans fats.

⚠ **Boost High Protein Nutritional Drinks**
33 g Net Carbs per can
  Contains added sugars.

FYI **Carnation Instant Breakfast No-Sugar-Added Shake Mix (Phases 3 & 4)**
12 g Net Carbs per packet
  Contains aspartame.

⚠ **Carnation Instant Breakfast Ready-to-Drink Shakes**
31 g Net Carbs per can
  Contains added sugars.

Carb Options Ready-to-Drink Shakes, Chocolate Delite, Creamy Vanilla (Phases 1-4)
2 g Net Carbs per can

FYI **Crystal Light Low-Cal Mix (Phases 1-4)**
0 g Net Carbs per cup
  Contains aspartame.

⚠ **Glucerna Shake**
26 g Net Carbs per can
  Contains added sugars.

**Slim-Fast Low Carb Shakes, Creamy Chocolate,
Vanilla Cream (Phases 1-4)**
2 g Net Carbs per can

⚠ **Slim-Fast Shakes, Original**
30–37 g Net Carbs per can, varies by flavor
  Contains added sugars.

⚠ **Westsoy Soy Shake, both flavors**
25-26 g Net Carbs per cup
  Contains added sugars.

SODAS

Nearly all diet sodas are sweetened with aspartame. Instead, look for brands that use sucralose (Splenda), and choose decaffeinated soda. Consuming too much caffeine can affect blood sugar, and it is also a diuretic, so you will need to drink 1 cup of water for every 8-ounce caffeinated beverage you drink.

And don't be misled by the name—tonic water is no tonic, but it is full of sugar—1 cup contains 22 grams of Net Carbs! Many diet tonic waters have 0 g Net Carbs per cup, but understand that they may also contain aspartame. If you're having trouble finding soft drinks that are acceptable, try combining seltzer with your favorite Atkins Sugar Free Flavored Syrup.

FYI **Diet Sodas, Seltzers, Tonic, most national brands (Phases 1-4)**
0 g Net Carbs per cup
May contain aspartame.

Boylan's Diet Soda, most flavors (Phases 1-4)
0 g Net Carbs per cup

Diet Rite Soda, most flavors (Phases 1-4)
0 g Net Carbs per cup

Hansen's Diet Soda, most flavors (Phases 1-4)
0 g Net Carbs per cup

Root 66 Diet Soda, most flavors (Phases 1-4)
0 g Net Carbs per cup

FLAVORED WATER

Watch out for sneaky sources of carbs in innocent-seeming waters. Infused waters use non-caloric sweeteners and flavorings and can be incorporated into a controlled-carb eating plan. However, some flavored waters contain sugar or other caloric sweeteners—so you might as well be drinking regular soda.

Arizona Infused Waters, most flavors (Phases 1-4)
0 g Net Carbs per cup

Fruit2O, all flavors (Phases 1-4)
0 g Net Carbs per cup

⚠ Gatorade Propel Fitness Water
3 g Net Carbs per cup
Contains added sugars.

Glaceau Fruit Water (Phases 1-4)
0 g Net Carbs per cup

Glaceau Smart Water (Phases 1-4)
0 g Net Carbs per cup

WATER, WATER EVERYWHERE . . .

Some flavored waters and those that have been infused with vitamins and minerals can be carb-free, refreshing drinks. But be careful—even within brands, some waters are acceptable while others are sky high in sugars and will drown you in carbs. Glaceau's Smart Waters, for example, average 0 grams Net Carbs per serving. But Glaceau's line known as Vitamin Water? A whopping 13 grams per 8 fluid ounces.

➤ ALCOHOLIC DRINKS ◄

Although you should not drink alcohol during the Induction phase of Atkins, when you move to Ongoing Weight Loss, you may begin to enjoy an occasional drink, if you so choose. But be selective—some types of alcoholic beverages have fewer grams of Net Carbs.

The body burns alcohol as a fuel before fat, so drinking alcohol can slow down the fat-burning process and postpone weight loss. Alcohol does not act as a carbohydrate so it will not interfere with burning fat in the same way that sugars and other carbohydrates do. However, if you add alcohol to your regimen and suddenly stop losing weight, discontinue your alcohol intake.

Please note: Even if you choose an alcoholic drink that is relatively low in carbs, alcoholic beverages should be consumed in moderation. That means, at most, one drink a day.

BEER

If you choose to drink beer, light and controlled-carb beers are your best bet. Some light beers are nearly as high as regular beers, however, so be sure to check labels.

Regular (Phases 3 & 4)
11–13 g Net Carbs per 12 ounces

Light (Phases 2-4)
• **Amstel Light** *5 g Net Carbs per 12 ounces*
• **Bud Light** *6.6 g Net Carbs per 12 ounces*
• **Labatt Blue Light** *8.3 g Net Carbs per 12 ounces*

Low-Carb (Phases 2-4)
• **Accel** *2.4 g Net Carbs per 12 ounces*
• **Martens** *2.1 g Net Carbs per 12 ounces*
• **Michelob Ultra** *2.6 g Net Carbs per 12 ounces*
• **Rhinebecker Extra Low Carbohydrate Brau**
  2.5 g Net Carbs per 12 ounces
• **Rock Green Light** *2.6 g Net Carbs per 12 ounces*

Non-Alcoholic (Phases 3 & 4)
12–15 g Net Carbs per 12 ounces

COCKTAIL MIXERS

When it comes to mixers for spirits, you're better off using sucralose-sweetened diet sodas and drinks. Use only mixers that contain no added sugars or fruit juices. In the later phases of Atkins, you may choose to use vegetable-based mixers. Likewise, avoid wine coolers, which typically weigh in with 32 grams of Net Carbs per 12 ounces.

Baja Bob's Crazy Caribe Pina Colada Mix!!
(Phases 2-4)
3 g Net Carbs per 4 ounces

AND . . . THEY'RE OFF!

The Great American controlled-carb beer race is on. Almost every brewery is competing to concoct the brew with the lowest carb count. The winner to date is Martens, with 2.1 grams of Net Carbs per 12-ounce serving. Accel, with 2.4 grams of Net Carbs per 12-ounce serving, comes in second. Following by a nose is Michelob Ultra (2.6 grams of Net Carbs).

How does that compare to *light* beers? Miller Lite comes in with 3.2 grams of Net Carbs, Milwaukee's Best with 3.5 grams, Coors Light with 4.4 grams, and Amstel Light and Corona Light trail the pack with 5 grams. And even more are expected in the coming year . . .

Baja Bob's Lean & Mean Bloody Mary Mix (Phases 2-4)
4 g Net Carbs per 4 ounces

Baja Bob's Sugar Free Margarita Mixes and Sweet and Sour Mix, Bottles (Phases 2-4)
1 g Net Carbs per ⅛ bottle

Baja Bob's Sugar Free Powdered Margarita Mixes (Phases 2-4)
3 g Net Carbs per 4 ounces

Bloody Mary Mix (Phases 3 & 4)
5–7 g Net Carbs per ½–¾ cup

Tomato Juice (Phases 3 & 4)
8 g Net Carbs per cup

WINE, CHAMPAGNE, AND SPIRITS

Desssert Wine, dry (Phases 2-4)
4 g Net Carbs per 3½ ounces

CHEERS?

Commercial cocktail mixes for margaritas and piña coladas typically add 30–50 grams of Net Carbs to your drink. That doesn't make for much of a Happy Hour. Indeed, the traditional versions of these drinks are unacceptable at any phase of Atkins. Ditto for cordials and sweet liquors.

But your favorite cocktails don't have to include high-sugar mixes. Look for sugar-free mixes from Baja Bob and toast your controlled-carb lifestyle with a Net Carb count of only 1–3 grams. Another plus: Their products use sucralose (Splenda).

Dessert Wine, sweet (Phases 3 & 4)
12 g Net Carbs per 3½ ounces

White Wine (Phases 2-4)
1 g Net Carbs per 3½ ounces

Red Wine (Phases 2-4)
2 g Net Carbs per 3½ ounces

Sherry, dry (Phases 2-4)
2 g Net Carbs per 2 ounces

Champagne (Phases 2-4)
2-4 g Net Carbs per 4 ounces

Hard Liquor, Bourbon, Gin, Rum, Vodka, any proof (Phases 2-4)
0 g Net Carbs per ounce

The Frozen Foods Aisle

Your supermarket's freezer section is one stop for pre-pared foods and ingredients that can help you maintain your controlled-carb lifestyle: frozen entrees (a perfect, speedy alternative to drive-thru), vegetables (buy bags, rather than boxes, and use just what you need), fruits no matter the season, even a few controlled-carb desserts. A few brands are vegetarian, too.

➤ FROZEN PRODUCTS ◄

ENTREES

Entrees that include rice, pasta and potatoes are going to be very high in carbohydrate, and some may include hydro-genated oils. Avoid all breaded meats, poultry and fish, too. Frozen French fries and onion rings are high in carbohydrate and hydrogenated oils.

FYI **Atkins Quick Quisine Pizza, Supreme, Smokehouse, Pepperoni (Phases 2-4)**
11 g Net Carbs per pizza
Contains nitrates.

Aaron's Best Glatt Kosher Turkey Schwarma (Phases 1-4)
3 g Net Carbs per 3 ounces

⚠ Jimmy Dean Original Sausage Links
0 g Net Carbs per 3 links
   Contains added sugars.

Jones Dairy Farm All-Natural 8 Little Sausages, Pork (Phases 1-4)
1 g Net Carbs per 3 links

⚠ Jones Dairy Farm Golden Brown Sausages, Mild
1 g Net Carbs per 3 links
   Contains added sugars.

⚠ Mike's Low Carb Gourmet Stir Fry Oriental Chicken Dinner
7 g Net Carbs per package
   Contains added sugars.

⚠ Mike's Low Carb Gourmet Chicken Breast Dinner
7 g Net Carbs per package
   Contains added sugars.

⚠ Mike's Low Carb Gourmet Chicken Marsala Dinner
9 g Net Carbs per package
   Contains added sugars.

⚠ Mike's Low Carb Gourmet Southern Jambalaya Dinner
11 g Net Carbs per package
   Contains added sugars.

⚠ Mike's Low Carb Gourmet Roasted Catfish Dinner
10 g Net Carbs per package
   Contains added sugars.

FYI Mrs. Paul's Marinated Shrimp Cajun (Phases 1-4)
2 g Net Carbs per 21 shrimp
   Contains MSG.

Mrs. Paul's Shrimp Scampi (Phases 1-4)
2 g Net Carbs per 25 shrimp

Mrs. Schreiber Chopped Liver Spread (Phases 2-4)
5 g Net Carbs per 2 ounces

Swift Premium Brown 'n Serve Sausage (Phases 1-4)
1 g Net Carbs per 3 links

Wampler Ground Turkey (Phases 1-4)
0 g Net Carbs per 4 ounces

Wampler Turkey Burger (Phases 1-4)
0 g Net Carbs per burger

FALSE FRIENDS

Grilled fish fillets, vegetable-based sausage links, a brand name like Healthy Choice—you'd expect them to be good for you, wouldn't you? Sometimes, things aren't as they seem. Boca Sausage Links, Gorton's Grilled Fish Fillets, and all Healthy Choice Meals contain hydrogenated oils.

SOUPS

Tabatchnick Barley & Mushroom, Low Sodium & No Added Sugars (Phases 3 & 4)
13 g Net Carbs per pouch

Tabatchnick Split Pea (Phases 3 & 4)
33 g Net Carbs per pouch

Tabatchnick Minestrone (Phases 3 & 4)
14 g Net Carbs per pouch

VEGETARIAN DISHES

See page 368 for additional frozen vegetarian options available at natural foods stores.

Boca Burgers Roasted Garlic (Phases 1-4)
2 g Net Carbs per patty

⚠ **Boca Burgers, All American Flame Grilled**
2 g Net Carbs per patty
   Contains trans fats.

Boca Burgers, Cheeseburger (Phases 1-4)
2 g Net Carbs per patty

Boca Burgers, Grilled Vegetable (Phases 1-4)
2 g Net Carbs per patty

⚠ **Boca Burgers, Roasted Onion**
3 g Net Carbs per patty
   Contains trans fats.

Boca Burgers, Original Vegan (Phases 1-4)
2 g Net Carbs per patty

⚠ **Boca Italian Sausage**
5 g Net Carbs per sausage
   Contains added sugars.

⚠ **Boca Smoked Sausage**
5 g Net Carbs per sausage
   Contains added sugars.

⚠ **Boca Bratwurst**
5 g Net Carbs per sausage
   Contains added sugars.

⚠ **Boca Chik'n Patties**
9 g Net Carbs per patty
   Contains trans fats.

⚠ **Boca Spicy Chik'n**
10 g Net Carbs per patty
   Contains trans fats.

⚠ **Boca Chik'n Nuggets**
15 g Net Carbs per 4 nuggets
   Contains trans fats.

Boca Meatless Ground Burger (Phases 1-4)
3 g Net Carbs per ½ cup

⚠ **Boca Breakfast Patties**
1 g Net Carbs per patty
   Contains trans fats.

⚠ **Boca Breakfast Links**
1 g Net Carbs per 2 links
   Contains added sugars and trans fats.

Boston Market Creamed Spinach (Phases 2-4)
7 g Net Carbs per ½ cup

⚠ **Gardenburger Diner Deluxe**
2 g Net Carbs per patty
   Contains added sugars.

FYI **Gardenburger Fire Roasted Vegetable**
(Phases 3 & 4)
14 g Net Carbs per patty
  Contains cornstarch.

Gardenburger Flame Grilled Hamburger Style
(Phases 1-4)
3 g Net Carbs per patty

Gardenburger Garden Vegan (Phases 3 & 4)
10 g Net Carbs per patty

Gardenburger Original (Phases 3 & 4)
13 g Net Carbs per patty

Gardenburger Sante Fe (Phases 3 & 4)
16 g Net Carbs per patty

⚠ **Gardenburger Savory Portabella**
14 g Net Carbs per patty
  Contains added sugars.

Gardenburger Veggie Medley (Phases 3 & 4)
15 g Net Carbs per patty

⚠ **Gardenburger Meatless Meatballs**
4 g Net Carbs per 6 meatballs
  Contains added sugars.

⚠ **Gardenburger Meatless Meatloaf**
8 g Net Carbs per slice
  Contains added sugars.

Gardenburger Buffalo Chik'n Wings (Phases 1-4)
3 g Net Carbs per 3 pieces

Gardenburger Meatless Breakfast Sausage (Phases 1-4)
0 g Net Carbs per patty

Golden Zucchini Pancakes (Phases 2-4)
7 g Net Carbs per pancake

Kohinoor dal Palek (Phases 3 & 4)
13 g Net Carbs per ⅓ package

Kohinoor Kashmiri Rajma (Phases 3 & 4)
17 g Net Carbs per package

Kohinoor Peshawari dal Makhani (Phases 3 & 4)
13 g Net Carbs per ⅓ package

⚠ **Mike's Low Carb Gourmet Eggplant Lasagna**
14 g Net Carbs per package
  Contains added sugars.

Morningstar Farms Better 'n Burgers (Phases 1-4)
3 g Net Carbs per patty

⚠ **Morningstar Farms Garden Veggie Patties**
5 g Net Carbs per patty
  Contains added sugars.

⚠ **Morningstar Farms Grillers**
3 g Net Carbs per patty
  Contains added sugars.

Morningstar Farm Harvest Burgers (Phases 1-4)
3 g Net Carbs per patty

⚠ **Yves Canadian Veggie Bacon**
2 g Net Carbs per 3 slices
  Contains added sugars.

Yves The Good Veggie Burger (Phases 1-4)
4 g Net Carbs per patty

⚠ Yves Le Good Dog
1 g Net Carbs per wiener
   Contains added sugars.

Yves Veggie "Neatballs" (Phases 1-4)
4 g Net Carbs per 5 meatballs

THE BIG CHILL: FREEZER TIPS

Make sure food is cold before you freeze it. This allows it to freeze faster and reduces the likelihood that your foods will develop freezer burn. Stop by the freezer aisle last. If food thaws, even briefly, before you put it in the freezer at home, its texture and flavor will suffer when you thaw it completely to cook. Your freezer temperature should remain constant at zero degrees Fahrenheit. Changes in temperature can ruin the food. If your controlled-carb ice cream forms ice crystals, this is an indication that your freezer's temperature is fluctuating.

For food safety, defrost foods in the refrigerator. Put meats and poultry on a plate to catch any liquid.

⚠ Yves Veggie Deli Slices
2 g Net Carbs per 3.5 slices
   Contains added sugars.

⚠ Yves Veggie Ground Round, Original
1 g Net Carbs per ⅓ cup
   Contains added sugars.

VEGETABLES

As with fresh vegetables, most frozen veggies are acceptable on Atkins—as long as what you're buying is *just* vegetables. Many frozen vegetables are swimming in sauces that can include starches; plus, butter-flavored and cheese-flavored sauces typically list partially hydrogenated vegetable oils as the first ingredient. Choose plain vegetables and cook them in broth for more flavor, then dress them with butter.

Even if you buy a box whose ingredients list touts only the vegetable, you may find that frozen vegetables are higher in Net Carbs than fresh ones. This is because frozen vegetables are always cooked, which frequently concentrates their nutrients.

Artichoke Hearts, most brands (Phases 1-4)
2 g Net Carbs per 12 pieces

Asparagus Spears, most brands (Phases 1-4)
2 g Net Carbs per 7 spears

Broccoli, most brands (Phases 1-4)
2 g Net Carbs per 2 spears or ¾ cup chopped

Brussels Sprouts, most brands (Phases 1-4)
4 g Net Carbs per ½ cup

Butternut Squash, most brands (Phases 3 & 4)
9 g Net Carbs per ½ cup

Carrots, most brands (Phases 3 & 4)
5 g Net Carbs per ½ cup

Cauliflower, most brands (Phases 1-4)
1 g Net Carbs per 4 pieces

Collard Greens, most brands (Phases 1-4)
0 g Net Carbs per ½ cup

Corn, most brands (Phases 3 & 4)
15 g Net Carbs per ½ cup

Corn, white, most brands (Phases 3 & 4)
12 g Net Carbs per ½ cup

Green Beans, most brands (Phases 1-4)
2 g Net Carbs per ½ cup cooked

Green Giant Green Beans with Almonds (Phases 2-4)
2 g Net Carbs per ½ cup cooked

⚠ **Green Giant Green Beans with Garlic Butter Sauce**
6 g Net Carbs per 1⅓ cup
   Contains added sugars.

Kale, most brands (Phases 1-4)
0 g Net Carbs per ½ cup

Lima Beans, baby, most brands (Phases 3 & 4)
15.5 g Net Carbs per ½ cup

Lima Beans, Fordhook, most brands (Phases 3 & 4)
14 g Net Carbs per ½ cup

Okra, most brands (Phases 1-4)
4 g Net Carbs per 9 pods

Peas, petite, most brands (Phases 3 & 4)
7 g Net Carbs per ⅔ cup

Peas, green, most brands (Phases 3 & 4)
8 g Net Carbs per ⅔ cup

Rutabaga, most brands (Phases 1-4)
1 g Net Carbs per ⅔ cup

Spinach, most brands (Phases 1-4)
2 g Net Carbs per 1 cup

Creamed Spinach, most brands (Phases 1-4)
6 g Net Carbs per ½ cup

Green Giant Cut-Leaf Spinach with Butter Sauce (Phases 1-4)
2 g Net Carbs per ½ cup

Squash, most brands (Phases 3 & 4)
9 g Net Carbs per ½ cup

Birds Eye Stir-Fry Vegetables (peppers and onions) (Phases 2-4)
4 g Net Carbs per cup

Birds Eye Stir-Fry Vegetables (broccoli, carrots, water chestnuts) (Phases 3 & 4)
5 g Net Carbs per cup

Succotash, most brands (Phases 3 & 4)
18 g Net Carbs per ⅔ cup

Green Giant Szechuan Vegetables (broccoli, water chestnuts, sugar snap peas, red bell peppers in Szechuan sauce) (Phases 3 & 4)
7 g Net Carbs per ¾ cup

Turnip Greens (with and without onions) (Phases 1-4)
0 g Net Carbs per ⅓ cup

FRUITS

Wondering why frozen fruit is higher in Net Carbs than fresh fruit is? When frozen foods thaw, ice crystals rupture the cell walls, so water escapes (this is why thawed meat has a watery liquid in the tray, for example). With less water, other nutrients, including carbohydrates, are concentrated. (See page 53 for fresh fruits.) Make sure the frozen fruit you purchase is unsweetened. Fruits may be sweetened; look for the words "unsweetened," "sugar-free," or "no-added-sugar" on the label and examine the ingredients list for sugar in all its forms including fruit juice concentrate.

Blackberries, most brands (Phases 2-4)
19 g Net Carbs per ¾ cup

Blueberries, most brands (Phases 2-4)
14 g Net Carbs per ¾ cup

Coconut Flakes, unsweetened (Phases 1-4)
1 g Net Carbs per 2 tablespoons
For a controlled-carb alternative to sweetened coconut flakes in the baking section, and for a speedy alternative to fresh coconut meat, look in the freezer for flat pouches of coconut flakes.

Mango Pulp (Phases 3 & 4)
8 g Net Carbs per ½ cup
It can be tricky to maneuver a knife around a fresh mango's large, oblong pit; frozen mango pulp, often stocked in flat pouches, is an easy alternative.

Maracuya Pulp (passion fruit) (Phases 3 & 4)
13 g Net Carbs per ½ cup
Passion fruit has a sweet yet tart flavor and is very aromatic; it's hard to find fresh passion fruit outside of markets

with a large Latin clientele, but you may find pulp, packed in flat pouches, in the freezer.

Mixed Berries, most varieties (Phases 2-4)
5 g Net Carbs per ½ cup

Mixed Fruits (grapes, melon balls) (Phases 3 & 4)
12 g Net Carbs per ⅔ cup

Papaya Chunks (Phases 3 & 4)
11 g Net Carbs per ⅔ cup

Peaches, most brands (Phases 3 & 4)
13 g Net Carbs per ⅔ cup

Raspberries, most brands (Phases 2-4)
10 g Net Carbs per ⅔ cup

Soursop (Phases 3 & 4)
17 g Net Carbs per ½ cup
   Soursops are from the same botanical family as cherimoyas (see page 62). The pulp is often used in ice cream and sherbet.

Strawberries, sliced, most brands (Phases 2-4)
13 g Net Carbs per ⅔ cup

Strawberries, whole, most brands (Phases 2-4)
5 g Net Carbs per ½ cup

Tamarind (Phases 3 & 4)
10 g Net Carbs per ½ cup
   Tamarind's sweet-tart pulp is common in Indian and Middle Eastern cooking; it is used to season curries, and it is an ingredient in Worcestershire sauce.

ICE CREAM AND DESSERTS

Atkins Endulge Super Premium Ice Cream Pints, Vanilla, Chocolate, Butter Pecan, Chocolate Peanut Butter Swirl, Vanilla Fudge Swirl, Chocolate Fudge Brownie, Vanilla Swiss Almond, Mint Chocolate Chip (Phases 2-4)
3 g Net Carbs per ½ cup

Atkins Endulge Super Premium Ice Cream Cups, Vanilla, Chocolate, Strawberry, Butter Pecan (Phases 2-4)
4 g Net Carbs per 4-ounce cup

FYI **Breyers No Sugar Added Light Ice Cream, French Vanilla (Phases 3 & 4)**
12 g Net Carbs per ½ cup
  Contains aspartame.

Breyers CarbSmart, Vanilla, Chocolate, Strawberry (Phases 2-4)
4 g Net Carbs per ½ cup

Blue Bunny Carb Freedom Frozen Dairy Dessert, Vanilla Bean (Phases 2-4)
2 g Net Carbs per ½ cup

Blue Bunny Carb Freedom Frozen Dairy Dessert, Double Strawberry (Phases 2-4)
4 g Net Carbs per ½ cup

⚠ Blue Bunny Carb Freedom Frozen Dairy Dessert, Butter Pecan, Chocolate Almond Fudge, Mint Chip
2-3 g Net Carbs per ½ cup
  Contains trans fats.

LeCarb Frozen Dessert, Vanilla, Chocolate Almond, Cinnamon, Homemade Vanilla, Strawberry (Phases 2-4)
3 g Net Carbs per ½ cup

⚠ LeCarb Frozen Dessert, Lemon
4 g Net Carbs per ½ cup
  Contains added sugars.

Dole No Sugar Added Fruit Juice Bars, all flavors (Phases 2-4)
5 g Net Carbs per bar

Edy's No Sugar Added Ice Cream, most flavors (Phases 3 & 4)
10 g Net Carbs per ½ cup

Tropicana No Sugar Added Fruit Juice Bars, all flavors (Phases 2-4)
1-2 g Net Carbs per bar

Welch's No Sugar Added Fruit Juice Bars, all flavors (Phases 2-4)
6 g Net Carbs per bar

NOVELTIES

Atkins Endulge Super Premium Ice Cream Bars, Chocolate Fudge (Phases 2-4)
2 g Net Carbs per bar

Atkins Endulge Super Premium Ice Cream Bars, Vanilla Fudge Swirl, Chocolate Fudge Swirl, Peanut Butter Fudge Swirl, Vanilla, Caramel Turtle Sundae, Butter Pecan (Phases 2-4)
3 g Net Carbs per bar

A COLD WAR:
ICE CREAM VS. FROZEN DESSERT

There's no doubt about it: We all scream for ice cream. Indeed, in 2000, U.S. production of ice cream and frozen desserts was more than 1.6 billion gallons, or approximately 23 quarts per person.

But did you know the cold, creamy stuff filling your pint may not be ice cream at all? In order to earn the name ice cream, federal law requires that a product contain at least 10 percent milk fat, before bulky ingredients are added, and weigh 4.5 pounds per gallon. To rise to the ranks of premium ice cream, it must have a butterfat content of at least 11 percent; super premium has a butterfat content of 16 percent. Super premium ice cream is denser and richer, and has a velvety texture. Items labeled "frozen desserts" do not meet these guidelines.

Blue Bunny Carb Freedom Novelties, Fudge Bar, Vanilla Bar (Phases 2-4)
2-3 g Net Carbs per bar

⚠ **Blue Bunny Carb Freedom Novelties, Almond Bar**
2 g Net Carbs per bar
  Contains trans fats.

CarbSmart Klondike Ice Cream Fudge Bar (Phases 2-4)
3 g Net Carbs per bar

CarbSmart Klondike Ice Cream Bar (Phases 2-4)
5 g Net Carbs per bar

LeCarb Frozen Bars, Chocolate, Strawberry (Phases 2-4)
3 g Net Carbs per bar

LeCarb Frozen Bars, Chocolate Almond, Lemon (Phases 2-4)
4 g Net Carbs per bar

WORST BITES: The frozen foods aisle has its fair share of Worst Bites. Here's the Hall of Shame:

- **Net Carb count is not enough:** Green Giant Green Bean Casserole doesn't seem like a bad choice; it has only 5 grams of Net Carbs per ⅔ cup. But the sauce contains hydrogenated oils.
- **Truth in packaging:** Birds Eye Broccoli, Carrots and Cauliflower with Cheese contains 5 grams of Net Carbs per ½ cup serving, and the box has a banner urging you to "Try for a Lunch or Quick Meal!" If you eat the whole bowl, you'll get 12.5 grams of Net Carbs . . . because there are 2.5 servings per package.
- **Ore-Ida Onion Rings have hydrogenated oils, and 27 grams of Net Carbs in a 4-ring serving.**
- **Pass on the pasta:** Green Giant Pasta Accents, as you might expect, contain a whopping 33 grams of Net Carbs per 2⅓ cup serving. It also contains partially hydrogenated oil, the fourth ingredient listed, after pasta, broccoli, and carrots.
- **Skip the sugar:** Unsweetened sliced strawberries have 13 grams of Net Carbs per ⅔ cup serving. Sliced with sugar? Almost three times as much—36 grams of Net Carbs per ⅔ cup.

PART 2:
THE NATURAL FOODS STORE

> ◄

The natural foods store is a terrific resource for obtaining controlled-carb, sugar-free, organic and trans fat-free foods, including many items that you won't find at your local supermarket. Most offer a greater variety of foods from smaller manufacturers, some of which specialize in reduced-carb items or aim to offer foods with particular health benefits. These stores also supply a range of bulk items, like nuts and unsweetened dried fruits, dried beans, soy and other vegetarian products, and often organic meats, wild fish and free-range poultry. Some nutrition stores also carry controlled-carb food products. (*Note: While there is some overlap among products available in supermarkets and natural foods stores, those that are also generally found in supermarkets, hypermarkets or club stores are listed in Part I.*)

Natural Foods

Although natural foods stores frequently carry a larger array of whole-grain baked goods and pastas and sugar-free foods than do supermarkets, you must not assume that everything "natural" fits within a controlled-carb lifestyle—or even a healthy one. Indeed, as is the case at the supermarket, you'll need to carefully examine food labels when you're searching the aisles here, too. Wheat-free products may be made with comparably high-carb grains, for example. White sugar and high-fructose corn syrup might not be on the ingredients list, but brown sugar, honey, barley syrup or rice syrup often take their place. And frozen treats made from soymilk are common offenders when it comes to added sugars.

On a positive note, natural foods are usually made with fewer starchy additives and although they might still be fairly high in carbohydrates, nibbles like snack foods, crackers, and cookies are usually (but not always) free of hydrogenated oils.

In addition, you're more likely to find organic produce, hormone-free and antibiotic-free meat and dairy products, as well as non-GMO foods. (See pages 371–373 for an explanation of these, and other, terms.)

➤ SLICED BREADS AND ROLLS ◄

For the most part, the breads in your natural foods store are far superior nutritional choices than those found in mainstream grocery stores. They almost always contain whole grains and whole-grain flours, and are frequently made without the added sugars, preservatives and hydrogenated oils you find in supermarket brands. They are also higher in fiber than breads made with bleached white flour or other refined grains.

Don't look for bread only in the bread aisle, though. Natural foods stores keep many of their breads refrigerated or frozen because whole grains are highly perishable in comparison to refined bakery products. These brands also lack, or contain minimal, preservatives. Atkins Bakery Ready-to-Eat Sliced Breads, Bagels and Rolls, for example, are often found in the freezer section.

In addition to whole-wheat breads, look for those made with brown rice, oats, spelt (a cereal grain), kamut (a variety of high-protein wheat), and millet. And keep an eye out for breads made from sprouted grains and legumes, sometimes called "manna" or "Ezekiel" breads. Sprouted grains are lower in carbohydrates, richer in nutrients and, some say, easier to digest. The sprouting process also chemically alters the gluten in grains, making these breads tolerable for some people with gluten sensitivities.

Finally, look for controlled-carb bread products from smaller bakeries and local or regional bread companies in your area. For example, Janet's Low Carb Bread, with 3 grams of Net Carbs per slice, is available in the New York Metropolitan area. As always, check the ingredients list for unacceptable ingredients and go over the Nutrition Facts panel carefully.

FYI **Atkins Bakery Ready-to-Eat Sliced Bread, Country White, Multigrain, Rye (Phases 1-4)**
3 g Net Carbs per slice
Contains enriched wheat flour.

FYI **Atkins Bakery Dinner Rolls (Phases 2-4)**
4 g Net Carbs per roll
  Contains enriched wheat flour.

FYI **Atkins Bakery Sandwich Rolls (Phases 2-4)**
5 g Net Carbs per roll
  Contains enriched wheat flour.

FYI **Atkins Bakery Hot Dog Rolls (Phases 2-4)**
5 g Net Carbs per roll
  Contains enriched wheat flour.

**⚠ Alvarado St. Bakery California Style Complete
Protein Bread**
12 g Net Carbs per slice
  Contains added sugars.

**Alvarado St. Bakery Sprouted Barley Bread
(Phases 3 & 4)**
15 g Net Carbs per slice

⚠ Alvarado St. Bakery Sprouted Multi-Grain Bread
13 g Net Carbs per slice
  Contains added sugars.

**Alvarado St. Bakery Sprouted Wheat Bread
(Phases 3 & 4)**
16 g Net Carbs per slice

**Alvarado St. Bakery Sprouted Wheat Rolls
(Phases 3 & 4)**
13 g Net Carbs per roll

⚠ Alvarado St. Bakery Sprouted Rye Seed
9 g Net Carbs per slice
  Contains added sugars.

Food for Life Low Carbohydrate Bread, Original
(Phases 1-4)
3 g Net Carbs per slice

Food for Life Low Carbohydrate Bread, Savory Herb
(Phases 1-4)
3 g Net Carbs per slice

French Meadow Bakery Kamut Bread
(Phases 3 & 4)
14 g Net Carbs per slice

French Meadow Bakery 100% Rye European Bread
(Phases 3 & 4)
19 g Net Carbs per slice

French Meadow Bakery 100% Rye with Flaxseed
(Phases 3 & 4)
19 g Net Carbs per slice

French Meadow Bakery 100% Rye with Sunflower
Seeds (Phases 3 & 4)
19 g Net Carbs per slice

French Meadow Bakery 100% Rye with Whole Grain
(Phases 3 & 4)
19 g Net Carbs per slice

French Meadow Bakery 100% Rye, Salt-Free Bread
(Phases 3 & 4)
19 g Net Carbs per slice

FYI **French Meadow Bakery Brown Rice Bread**
(Phases 3 & 4)
11 g Net Carbs per slice
   Contains flour.

French Meadow Bakery Sunflower & Flax Bread (Phases 3 & 4)
15 g Net Carbs per slice

French Meadow Bakery Healthseed 100% Rye Bread (Phases 3 & 4)
16 g Net Carbs per slice

French Meadow Bakery Healthseed Spelt Bread (Phases 3 & 4)
10 g Net Carbs per slice

FYI **French Meadow Bakery Healthy Hemp, Sprouted (Phases 2-4)**
7 g Net Carbs per slice
  Contains flour.

FYI **French Meadow Bakery Men's Bread (Phases 2-4)**
5 g Net Carbs per slice
  Contains flour.

French Meadow Bakery Millet Bread (Phases 3 & 4)
18 g Net Carbs per slice

French Meadow Bakery Peasant Rolls (Phases 3 & 4)
17 g Net Carbs per roll

French Meadow Bakery Spelt Bread (Phases 3 & 4)
12 g Net Carbs per slice

French Meadow Bakery Spelt Bread with Wild Rice (Phases 3 & 4)
22 g Net Carbs per slice

French Meadow Bakery Spelt Cinnamon Raisin Bread (Phases 3 & 4)
16 g Net Carbs per slice

French Meadow Bakery Spelt Pizza Crust (Phases 3 & 4)
13 g Net Carbs per ¼ of 8-inch crust

**French Meadow Bakery Sprouted Whole Wheat Bread
(Phases 3 & 4)**
12 g Net Carbs per slice

French Meadow Bakery Summer Bread (Phases 3 & 4)
14 g Net Carbs per slice

FYI French Meadow Bakery Woman's Bread with Soy
Isoflavones (Phases 2-4)
7 g Net Carbs per slice
  Contains flour.

**Genuine Bavarian Organic Multi-Grain Bread
(Phases 3 & 4)**
14 g Net Carbs per slice

**Genuine Bavarian Organic Whole Rye/Oat Bread
(Phases 3 & 4)**
15 g Net Carbs per slice

⚠ LifeStyle Low Carb Bread
4 g Net Carbs per slice
  Contains added sugars.

O' So Lo Lo-Carb Rollz, Original (Phases 1-4)
3 g Net Carbs per roll

O' So Lo Lo-Carb Rollz, Pumpernickel (Phases 1-4)
3 g Net Carbs per roll

O' So Lo Lo-Carb Rollz, Sourdough (Phases 1-4)
3 g Net Carbs per roll

O' So Lo Lo-Carb Sweet Rollz, Banana Walnut (Phases 2-4)
3 g Net Carbs per roll

O' So Lo Lo-Carb Sweet Rollz, Cinnamon Raisin (Phases 1-4)
3 g Net Carbs per roll

⚠ Rudi's Organic Bakery Bread, Low-Carb, Low-Carb Herb
4 g Net Carbs per slice
   Contains added sugars.

Sunnyvale Bakery Carrot Raisin Sprouted Bread (Phases 3 & 4)
20 g Net Carbs per slice

Sunnyvale Bakery Date Cinnamon (Phases 3 & 4)
20 g Net Carbs per serving

Sunnyvale Bakery Fruit Almond Bread (Phases 3 & 4)
21 g Net Carbs per slice

Sunnyvale Bakery Original Sprouted Bread (Phases 3 & 4)
20 g Net Carbs per slice

Sunnyvale Bakery Raisin Bread (Phases 3 & 4)
21 g Net Carbs per slice

Sunnyvale Bakery Sunseed Sprouted Bread (Phases 3 & 4)
18 g Net Carbs per slice

Suzie's Kamut Breadsticks, Sesame (Phases 3 & 4)
16 g Net Carbs per 2 breadsticks

The Baker Low Carb Bran (Phases 2-4)
4 g Net Carbs per ounce

The Baker Low Carb Flax (Phases 2-4)
4 g Net Carbs per ounce

➤ BAGELS, MUFFINS, AND TORTILLAS ◄

While sliced breads are keeping up with the needs of those following a controlled-carb lifestyle, bagels, muffins and tortillas are a little behind the times. Most ready-to-eat varieties are still made with bleached flour and/or sugar and tend to be very high in Net Carbs. In later phases, your selection will be broader, thanks to tortillas made with whole-wheat flour and other whole grains, as well as the growing number of low-carb bagels and muffins.

Seek out chapati, an unleavened bread from India, which is made from whole-wheat flour and water. It can be used as you would tortillas.

FYI **Atkins Bakery Tortillas (Phases 2-4)**
5 g Net Carbs per tortilla
Contains enriched wheat flour.

FYI **Atkins Bakery Ready-to-Eat Pre-Sliced Bagels, Plain (Phases 2-4)**
7 g Net Carbs per bagel
Contains enriched wheat flour.

FYI **Atkins Bakery Ready-to-Eat Pre-Sliced Bagels, Onion (Phases 2-4)**
8 g Net Carbs per bagel
Contains enriched wheat flour.

FYI Atkins Bakery Ready-to-Eat Pre-Sliced Bagels, Cinnamon Raisin (Phases 2-4)
9 g Net Carbs per bagel
  Contains enriched wheat flour.

Alvarado St. Bakery Sprouted Wheat Tortillas, Burrito Size (Phases 3 & 4)
24 g Net Carbs per tortilla

Alvarado St. Bakery Sprouted Wheat Tortillas, Fajita Size (Phases 3 & 4)
21 g Net Carbs per tortilla

Food for Life Sprouted Grain Tortillas, Ezekiel 4:9 (Phases 3 & 4)
19 g Net Carbs per tortilla

Garden of Eatin' Chapati (Phases 3 & 4)
18 g Net Carbs per chapati

Garden of Eatin' Blue Corn Tortillas (Phases 3 & 4)
20 g Net Carbs per 2 tortillas

Garden of Eatin' Whole Wheat Tortillas (Phases 3 & 4)
20 g Net Carbs per tortilla

O' So Lo Lo-Carb Muffins, Blueberry (Phases 2-4)
5 g Net Carbs per muffin

O' So Lo Lo-Carb Muffins, Chocolate, Peanut Butter (Phases 2-4)
4 g Net Carbs per muffin

O' So Lo Lo-Carb Muffins, Apple Spice, Banana, Vanilla (Phases 1-4)
3 g Net Carbs per muffin

➤ CEREAL ◄

COLD CEREAL

Cereals are high in carbs for two reasons: Corn, oats and wheat, the most common cereal grains, are dense in carbohydrates, and cold cereals almost always contain added sweeteners.

You won't necessarily see the words *sugar* or even *corn syrup* on boxes in a natural foods store. Instead, you'll see terms such as evaporated cane juice, fruit juice concentrate, molasses, honey or malt extract. Don't be lured in by these natural, homey sounding terms—they're just aliases for sugar.

Most cereals—including those health food staples muesli and granola—have Net Carb counts of between 20 and 50 grams per serving (serving sizes aren't uniform among the brands). Aside from controlled-carb cereals such as Atkins Morning Start Cereals, the top options are plain, whole-grain cereals that contain no additional sugars. The same holds true for hot cereals: When your carb threshold allows it, your best bet is old-fashioned rolled or steel-cut oats or another whole-grain cereal.

Atkins Morning Start Cereal, Crunchy Almond Crisp (Phases 2-4)
3 g Net Carbs per ⅔ cup

Atkins Morning Start Cereal, Blueberry Bounty with Almonds (Phases 2-4)
4 g Net Carbs per ⅔ cup

Atkins Morning Start Cereal, Banana Nut Harvest (Phases 2-4)
5 g Net Carbs per ⅔ cup

⚠ Arrowhead Mills Organic Oat Bran Flakes
11 g Net Carbs per cup
   Contains added sugars.

Arrowhead Mills Organic Nature O's Cereal
(Phases 3 & 4)
23 g Net Carbs per cup

⚠ **Arrowhead Mills Perfect Harvest Cereal**
20 g Net Carbs per cup
  Contains added sugars.

Arrowhead Mills Puffed Cereal, Corn, Millet, Wheat
(Phases 3 & 4)
10 g Net Carbs per cup

Arrowhead Mills Puffed Kamut Cereal (Phases 3 & 4)
9 g Net Carbs per cup

Arrowhead Mills Puffed Rice Cereal (Phases 3 & 4)
4 g Net Carbs per cup

Arrowhead Mills Shredded Wheat Cereal
(Phases 3 & 4)
32 g Net Carbs per cup

⚠ **Barbara's Bakery Puffins, Original**
18 g Net Carbs per ¾ cup
  Contains added sugars.

Barbara's Bakery 100% Whole Wheat No Sugar Added
Shredded Wheat (Phases 3 & 4)
26 g Net Carbs per 2 biscuits

Bob's Red Mill Apple Cinnamon Grains Cereal
(Phases 3 & 4)
19 g Net Carbs per ¼ cup

Bob's Red Mill 8-Grain Wheatless Cereal
(Phases 3 & 4)
18 g Net Carbs per ¼ cup

Bob's Red Mill 5-Grain Rolled Cereal (Phases 3 & 4)
20 g Net Carbs per ⅓ cup

Bob's Red Mill Grains & Nuts Cereal (Phases 3 & 4)
17 g Net Carbs per ¼ cup

**Bob's Red Mill Muesli Old Country Style
(Phases 3 & 4)**
16 g Net Carbs per ¼ cup

**CarbSense MiniCarb Granola, Apple Cinnamon
(Phases 2-4)**
4 g Net Carbs per ½ cup

Keto Crisp Cereal, Original, Cocoa (Phases 2-4)
3 g Net Carbs per ⅔ cup

**FYI Keto Frosted Flakes, Classic, Apple Cinnamon,
Honey Nut (Phases 2-4)**
3 g Net Carbs per ¼ cup
   Contains potato starch.

⚠ Protein Plus
21 g Net Carbs per ⅔ cup
   Contains added sugars.

Simply Fiber (Phases 3 & 4)
17 g Net Carbs per cup

Uncle Sam Cold Cereal (Phases 3 & 4)
28 g Net Carbs per cup

HOT CEREAL

Ancient Harvest Quinoa Flakes (Phases 3 & 4)
20.4 g Net Carbs per ⅓ cup dry

**Arrowhead Mills 4 Grain Plus Flax Hot Cereal
(Phases 3 & 4)**
19 g Net Carbs per ¼ cup dry

Arrowhead Mills Oat Flakes Hot Cereal (Phases 3 & 4)
19 g Net Carbs per ⅓ cup dry

**Arrowhead Mills Organic Oat Bran Hot Cereal
(Phases 3 & 4)**
17 g Net Carbs per ⅓ cup dry

**Arrowhead Mills Instant Oatmeal, Original
(Phases 3 & 4)**
17 g Net Carbs per packet

**Arrowhead Mills Instant Oatmeal, Cinnamon Raisin
Almond (Phases 3 & 4)**
21 g Net Carbs per packet

**Arrowhead Mills Old-Fashioned Oatmeal
(Phases 3 & 4)**
19 g Net Carbs per ⅓ cup dry

**Arrowhead Mills Seven Grain Hot Cereal
(Phases 3 & 4)**
22 g Net Carbs per ⅓ cup dry

**Arrowhead Mills Steel Cut Oats Hot Cereal
(Phases 3 & 4)**
19 g Net Carbs per ¼ cup dry

**Bob's Red Mill 5-Grain Rolled Hot Cereal
(Phases 3 & 4)**
20 g Net Carbs per ⅓ cup dry

**Bob's Red Mill Organic Creamy Buckwheat Cereal
(Phases 3 & 4)**
18 g Net Carbs per ⅛ cup dry

Bob's Red Mill Right Stuff Hot Cereal (Phases 3 & 4)
23 g Net Carbs per ¼ cup dry

Bob's Red Mill Triticale Cereal (Phases 3 & 4)
19 g Net Carbs per ¼ cup dry

**CarbSense Instant Hot Cereal, Country Spice
(Phases 2-4)**
3 g Net Carbs per ½ cup dry

**CarbSense Instant Hot Cereal, Roasted Hazelnut
(Phases 2-4)**
3 g Net Carbs per ½ cup dry

**CarbSense MiniCarb Instant Hot Cereal, Milk
Chocolate (Phases 2-4)**
4 g Net Carbs per ½ cup dry

**Country Choice Organic Instant Oatmeal, Regular
(Phases 3 & 4)**
16 g Net Carbs per packet

**Erewhon Instant Oatmeal, Organic, with Added Oat
Bran (Phases 3 & 4)**
21 g Net Carbs per packet

**Keto Hot Cereal, Old-Fashioned Oatmeal, Apple
Cinnamon, Banana Nut, Blueberry & Crème,
Strawberry & Crème (Phases 2-4)**
3 g Net Carbs per 2 scoops

Uncle Sam Instant Oatmeal (Phases 3 & 4)
19 g Net Carbs per packet

➤ CHEESE SUBSTITUTES ◄

The natural foods store is a good place to find non-dairy substitutes for cow's and goat's milk-based cheeses. Made of soy or rice, they are typically very low in carbs, ranging from 0 grams of Net Carbs per ounce to 3 grams of Net Carbs per slice. You may need to experiment a little to find one with the qualities you're looking for—say, meltability—and a taste and texture that appeals to you.

Soy Moon Real Gourmet Soy Cheese, Soy Gouda, Soy Provolone (Phases 1-4)
1 g Net Carbs per ounce

Soy Moon Real Gourmet Soy Cheese, Soy Mozzarella (Phases 1-4)
0 g Net Carbs per ounce

Soya Kaas, Jalapeño Mexi-Kaas (Phases 1-4)
1 g Net Carbs per ounce

Soya Kaas, Mild Cheddar Style, Garlic & Herb (Phases 1-4)
0 g Net Carbs per serving

Soya Kaas, Mozzarella Style (Phases 1-4)
0 g Net Carbs per serving

Tofu Rella Mozzarella Slices (Phases 1-4)
1 g Net Carbs per slice

Tofu Rella, Cheddar Flavor (Phases 1-4)
1 g Net carbs per ounce

🔺 **Tofutti Slice, Mozzarella, American**
2 g Net Carbs per slice
  Contains trans fats.

Yves The Good Slice, American Style (Phases 1-4)
0 g Net Carbs per serving

Yves The Good Slice, Mozzarella Style (Phases 1-4)
0 g Net Carbs per serving

Yves The Good Slice, Jalapeño-Jack (Phases 1-4)
0 g Net Carbs per slice

Yves The Good Slice, Cheddar Style (Phases 1-4)
1 g Net Carbs per slice

➤ CRACKERS, CRISPBREADS, ◄ AND BREADSTICKS

If there is one aisle in which you're likely to find more options at the natural foods stores, it's the cracker department. Instead of bleached white flour and sugar, you will find whole-grain products. Hydrogenated oils are ubiquitous in supermarket-brand crackers, but crackers found in the natural foods store tend to be free of them. Natural brands prove that you truly don't need this dangerous fat to make crispy, tasty, shelf-stable crackers!

The not-so-good news is you won't find most of these healthier crackers to be much lower in carbs. There are a few controlled-carb standouts, however, so scan your shelves carefully. If you can find them, brands specializing in controlled-carb crackers will be much lower overall.

FYI **Annie's Cheddar Bunnies (Phases 3 & 4)**
18 g Net Carbs per 7 crackers
   Contains wheat flour.

FYI **Barbara's Bakery Cheese Bites (Phases 3 & 4)**
20 g Net Carbs per 22 crackers
  Contains wheat flour.

⚠ Barbara's Bakery Wheatines, Original
11 g Net Carbs per 4 crackers/1 sheet
  Contains added sugars.

**Bisca Organic Mini Water Crackers, Sesame
(Phases 3 & 4)**
12 g Net Carbs per 8 crackers

Bran-a-Crisp (Phases 2-4)
4 g Net Carbs per cracker

**Cheeters Diet Treats Crackers, most flavors
(Phases 2-4)**
1 g Net Carb per 3 crackers

**Edward & Sons Brown Rice Snaps, Cheddar
(Phases 3 & 4)**
13 g Net Carbs per 8 crackers

**Edward & Sons Brown Rice Snaps, Tamari Sesame
(Phases 3 & 4)**
11 g Net Carbs per 8 crackers

**Edward & Sons Brown Rice Snaps, Toasted Onion
(Phases 3 & 4)**
13 g Net Carbs per 8 crackers

**Edward & Sons Brown Rice Snaps, Unsalted Plain
(Phases 3 & 4)**
12 g Net Carbs per 8 crackers

Edward & Sons Brown Rice Snaps, Vegetable (Phases 3 & 4)
12 g Net Carbs per 8 crackers

⚠ Frookie All Natural Wheat and Rye Snack Crackers
15 g Net Carbs per 13 crackers
  Contains added sugars.

GG Scandinavian Bran Crispbread (Phases 2-4)
0 g Net Carbs per slice

⚠ Health Valley Garden Herb Natural Wheat Crackers
9 g Net Carbs per 6 crackers
  Contains added sugars.

Heavenly Desserts Sesame Crackers (Phases 2-4)
3 g Net Carbs per cracker

Hol-Grain Crackers, Brown Rice, Brown Rice with Onion and Garlic, No Salt Brown Rice (Phases 3 & 4)
13 g Net Carbs per 7 crackers

Hol-Grain Crackers, Whole Wheat (Phases 3 & 4)
11 g Net Carbs per 8 crackers

Orgran Crispbreads, Rice & Garden Herb (Phases 2-4)
9 g Net Carbs per 2 slices

Orgran Crispbreads, Salsa Corn (Phases 3 & 4)
16 g Net Carbs per 4 slices

Quilts Dark Rye Crackers (Phases 2-4)
9 g Net Carbs per 2 crackers

Quilts Light Rye Crackers (Phases 2-4)
8 g Net Carbs per 2 crackers

San-J Black Sesame Rice Crackers (Phases 3 & 4)
16 g Net Carbs per 5 crackers

San-J Sesame Brown Rice Crackers (Phases 3 & 4)
18 g Net Carbs per 5 crackers

San-J Tamari Brown Rice Crackers (Phases 3 & 4)
25 g Net Carbs per 6 crackers

Suzie's Kamut Breadsticks, Sesame (Phases 3 & 4)
16 g Net Carbs per 2 breadsticks

Suzie's Kamut Flatbreads, Sesame (Phases 3 & 4)
17 g Net Carbs per 3 flatbreads

➤ SNACK FOODS ◄

SALTY, CRUNCHY SNACKS

They may be all-natural, organic, wheat-free, trans fat-free, and non-GMO, but most chips, crisps, sticks, pretzels, and puffs still have between 18 and 22 grams of Net Carbs per ounce. Soy crisps and chips are a notch lower than snacks made with flour, cornmeal, or potato flour; they tend to be about 12 grams of Net Carbs per ounce (except the barbecue flavor versions, which are about 17). Soy nuts, which are roasted soybeans, are a great salty snack at just 4 grams of Net Carbs per ½ cup, on average. Plus they offer up 5 grams of fiber and 14 grams of protein.

Another terrific crunchy snack is good old-fashioned popcorn. One cup of air-popped popcorn has a mere 5 grams of Net Carbs and 1 gram of fiber. Microwaveable popcorn tends to have more carbs and most, whether described as "natural" or not, contain hydrogenated oils.

Baja Bob's Soy Munchables, Cool Ranch, Jalapeño (Phases 1-4)
3 g Net Carbs per ounce

FYI **Baja Bob's Soy Munchables, Italian (Phases 1-4)**
3 g Net Carbs per ounce
  Contains MSG.

Barbara's Bakery Cheese Puffs, Original, Jalapeño (Phases 3 & 4)
16 g Net Carbs per 1½ cups

Barbara's Bakery Cheese Puff Bakes, Original, White Cheddar (Phases 3 & 4)
13 g Net Carbs per 1½ cups

CarbFit Soy Nuts, Salted, Red Hot (Phases 2-4)
6 g Net Carbs per ⅓ cup

⚠ CarbFit Soy Twirls, Cool Ranch, Nacho Cheese
5 g Net Carbs per ounce
  Contains added sugars.

CarbFit Tortilla Chips (Phases 2-4)
5 g Net Carbs per ounce

Eden Brown Rice Chips (Phases 3 & 4)
19 g Net Carbs per 50 chips

Glad Corn A-Maizing Corn Snack, Original (Phases 3 & 4)
15 g Net Carbs per ounce

⚠ Glenny's Soy Crisps, Apple Cinnamon
9 g Net Carbs per ounce
  Contains added sugars.

Glenny's Soy Crisps, Lightly Salted, Salt & Pepper, New Cheddar (Phases 3 & 4)
8 g Net Carbs per ounce

⚠ **Glenny's Soy Crispy Wispys, Sour Cream and Onion**
6 g Net Carbs per 14 grams
   Contains added sugars.

Glenny's Soy Crispy Wispys, White Cheddar, Nacho Cheese (Phases 2-4)
6 g Net Carbs per 14 grams

⚠ **Glenny's Soy Crispy Wispys, Zesty Veggie**
7 g Net Carbs per 14 grams
   Contains added sugars.

Glenny's Veggie Chips, Mixed Veggie (Phases 2-4)
6 g Net Carbs per 12 chips

⚠ **Hain Soy Munchies, Caramel**
8 g Net Carbs per 7 pieces
   Contains added sugars.

⚠ **Hain Soy Munchies, Ranch**
7 g Net Carbs per 9 pieces
   Contains added sugars.

Hain Soy Munchies, White Cheddar (Phases 2-4)
5 g Net Carbs per 9 pieces

Happy Herbert's Ancient Grains Kamut Snack Sticks (Phases 3 & 4)
12 g Net Carbs per 26 pieces

FYI **Happy Herbert's Ancient Grains Sesame Snack Sticks (Phases 3 & 4)**
11 g Net Carbs per 25 pieces
  Contains wheat flour.

Happy Herbert's Ancient Grains Spelt Snack Sticks (Phases 3 & 4)
11 g Net Carbs per 26 pieces

FYI **Happy Herbert's Ancient Grains Wild Rice Snack Sticks (Phases 3 & 4)**
15 g Net Carbs per 22 pieces
  Contains wheat flour.

Happy Herbert's Ancient Grains Spelt Mini Pretzels (Phases 3 & 4)
20 g Net Carbs per 16 pretzels

Happy Herbert's All Natural Popcorn (Phases 2-4)
8 g Net Carbs per 3 cups

Happy Herbert's White Cheddar Cheese Popcorn (Phases 3 & 4)
8 g Net Carbs per 2½ cups

Happy Herbert's Zany Corn (Phases 3 & 4)
16 g Net Carbs per ½ cup

Just The Cheese, White Cheddar, Sour Cream & Onion, Cool Ranch, Lo-Salt White Cheddar, Nacho, Pizza (Phases 1-4)
1 g Net Carbs per bar or 1-ounce serving

Kettle Tortilla Chips, Blue Corn, Five Grain Yellow Corn (Phases 3 & 4)
16 g Net Carbs per ounce

Keto Tortilla Chips, Classic Corn, Cool Ranch, Nacho Cheese (Phases 2-4)
4 g Net Carbs per ounce

Kettle Tortilla Chips, Sesame Rye with Caraway (Phases 3 & 4)
15 g Net Carbs per ounce

Little Bear Lite Cheddar Puffs (Phases 3 & 4)
18 g Net Carbs per 2 cups

Nature's Hilights Lite 'n Crispy Rice Snacks (Phases 2-4)
7 g Net Carbs per 6 sticks

Pumpkorn, Original, Chili, Curry (Phases 2-4)
2 g Net Carbs per ⅓ cup

Quality Green Sesame Crunch Roasted Sesame Seeds Snack (Phases 2-4)
2 g Net Carbs per 4 bars

Skinny Soy Chips, Lightly Salted (Phases 3 & 4)
9 g Net Carbs per ounce

Skinny Soy Chips, Wasabi Ginger (Phases 3 & 4)
10 g Net Carbs per ounce

COOKIES

When you're purchasing controlled-carb cookies, be extra careful—a large number of them, including those from companies specializing in controlled-carb foods, are nutritional wolves in sheep's clothing. Indeed, those that are very low in grams of Net Carbs are often hiding unacceptable ingredients, from sweeteners to white flour to hydrogenated oils.

Atkins Endulge Chewy Chocolate Chip Cookie Bites (Phases 2-4)
5 g Net Carbs per serving

⚠️ **CarbFit Cookies, Almond, Chocolate Chip**
9 g Net Carbs per 2 cookies
   Contains added sugars.

⚠️ **CarbFit Cookies, Peanut Butter**
8 g Net Carbs per 2 cookies
   Contains added sugars.

⚠️ **Carborite Cookies, Shortbread, Chocolate Chip**
3 g Net Carbs per cookie
   Contains trans fats.

⚠️ **Carborite Peanut Butter Cookies**
4 g Net Carbs per cookie
   Contains trans fats.

Glenny's Slim Carb Soy Fudgies, Brownie Cookies, Chocolate Raspberry (Phases 1-4)
2 g Net Carbs per ounce

Glenny's Slim Carb Soy Fudgies, Mint Fudge, Fancy Fudge (Phases 3 & 4)
3 g Net Carbs per ounce

FYI **Gol D Lites Sugar-Free Belgian Waffles (Phases 2–4)**
7 g Net Carbs per waffle
   Contains wheat flour.

Heavenly Desserts Meringues, most flavors (Phases 1-4)
0 g Net Carbs per cookie

Keto Italian-Style Biscotti, all flavors (Phases 2-4)
4 g Net Carbs per cookie

Lite Harvest Low Carb Enchantments, Peanut Butter Chocolate Chunk (Phases 2-4)
3 g Net Carbs per cookie

Low Carb Creations Cookies, Chocolate Chip, Coconut, Snickerdoodle, Lemon, Peanut Butter (Phases 2-4)
2 g Net Carbs per cookie

⚠️ **Mi-Del Snaps, Vanilla, Chocolate, Ginger, Lemon**
20-21 g Net Carbs per 5 cookies
   Contains added sugars.

Pure De-lite Oven-Baked High-Protein Cookies, Chocolate Fudge (Phases 2-4)
0 g Net Carbs

Pure De-lite Oven-Baked High-Protein Cookies, Peanut Butter Crunch (Phases 2-4)
0 g Net Carbs

The Smarter Carb, Almond Chip Biscotti (Phases 2-4)
0 g Net Carbs per 3 cookies

The Smarter Carb, Chocolate Covered Meringues (Phases 2-4)
0 g Net Carbs per 3 cookies

The Smarter Carb, Chocolate Covered Biscotti (Phases 2-4)
1 g Net Carbs per 3 cookies

SoyBite 1-Carb Cookies, Coconut (Phases 2-4)
1 g Net Carbs per 1½ cookies

CANDY AND SWEETS

The burgeoning market for controlled-carb candy is a testament to our love of all things sweet. These items manage to keep the carbs down because they contain sugar alcohols, a kind of indigestible sweetener. Sounds good, doesn't it? Unfortunately, sugar alcohols can produce a laxative effect in some individuals, so tread slowly into this area until you figure out your tolerance. Also watch out for hydrogenated oils and added sugar, which abound here.

Atkins Endulge Bits Candies (Phases 2-4)
2 g Net Carbs per bar

Atkins Endulge Caramel Nut Chew (Phases 2-4)
2 g Net Carbs per bar

Atkins Endulge Double Milk Chocolate, Double Milk Chocolate Crunch Candy Bar (Phases 2-4)
2 g Net Carbs per bar

Atkins Endulge Peanut Caramel Cluster (Phases 2-4)
1 g Net Carbs per bar

FYI **Atkins Endulge Wafer Crisp Bars, Mint, Peanut Butter, Chocolate Crème, Vanilla Crème (Phases 2-4)**
4 g Net Carbs per bar 2-stick pak
Contains wheat flour.

Atkins Endulge Peanut Butter Cups (Phases 2-4)
2 g Net Carbs per 3-cup package

Atkins Endulge Chocolate Candy Bars, Chocolate, Chocolate Crunch (Phases 2-4)
2 g Net Carbs per bar

Carborite At Last! Candy Bars, Chocolate Almond, Chocolate Mint (Phases 2-4)
1 g Net Carbs per bar

Carborite At Last! Candy Bars, Chocolate Crisp (Phases 2-4)
2 g Net Carbs per bar

⚠ **Carborite At Last! Chocolate Bars, Peanut Butter, Chocolate Truffle**
1 g Net Carbs per bar
  Contains trans fats.

⚠ **Carborite At Last! Chocolate Covered Peanuts**
3 g Net Carbs per 35 grams
  Contains trans fats.

⚠ **Carborite Caramel Nougat Bar**
0 g Net Carbs per bar
  Contains trans fats.

⚠ **Carborite Crispy Caramel Bar**
0 g Net Carbs per bar
  Contains trans fats.

Carborite Chocolate Bars, Chocolate Almond, Milk Chocolate, Chocolate Mint (Phases 2-4)
0 g Net Carbs per bar

Carborite Chocolate Bars, Chocolate Crisp (Phases 2-4)
1 g Net Carbs per bar

⚠ **Carborite Chocolate Bars, Chocolate Peanut Butter**
1 g Net Carbs per bar
  Contains trans fats.

Carborite Chocolate Bars, Dark Chocolate (Phases 2-4)
0 g Net Carbs per bar

Carborite Chocolate Covered Almonds (Phases 2-4)
2 g Net Carbs per 40 grams

⚠️ **Carborite Chocolate Covered Peanuts**
3 g Net Carbs per 9 pieces
   Contains trans fats.

Carborite Gummy Bears (Phases 2-4)
0 g Net Carbs per 17 pieces

Carborite Jelly Beans (Phases 2-4)
3 g Net Carbs per 26 pieces

Carborite Peanut Butter Cup (Phases 2-4)
0 g Net Carbs

⚠️ **Carborite Pecan Caramel Cluster**
1 g Net Carbs per 35 grams
   Contains trans fats.

Carborite Sour Citrus Slices (Phases 2-4)
0 g Net Carbs per 15 pieces

⚠️ **Carborite Toffee Chews, Chocolate, Vanilla**
3 g Net Carbs per 40 grams
   Contains trans fats.

CarbSlim Bites, both flavors (Phases 2-4)
0 g Net Carbs per box

Carbwatchers Chocolate Bar, most flavors (Phases 2-4)
8 g Net Carbs per bar

Doctor's CarbRite Diet Chocolate-Covered Brown Rice Cakes (Phases 2-4)
9 g Net Carbs per cake

Doctor's CarbRite Diet Sugar-Free Chocolate Bar, most flavors (Phases 2-4)
0 g Net Carbs per bar

Gol D Lites Chocolate-Coated Marshmallow Bar (Phases 1-4)
1 g Net Carbs per bar

Gol D Lites Sugar-Free Marshmallows (Phases 1-4)
0 g Net Carbs per ⅓ bag

Ketogenics Low Carb Chocolate Bars, Chocolate Crisp, Chocolate Almond, Chocolate Peanut Butter (Phases 2-4)
1-2 g Net Carbs per bar

La Nouba Chocolate Bars, Dark, Milk (Phases 2-4)
4 g Net Carbs per bar

La Nouba Marshmallows (Phases 1-4)
0 g Net Carbs per serving

Low Carb Creations Gourmet Cheesecake, most flavors (Phases 2-4)
1 g Net Carbs per 1 ounce

Low Carb Creations Gourmet Soft Brittle (Phases 2-4)
2 g Net Carbs per piece

⚠ **Pure De-lite Caramel, Caramel Crisp, Caramel Nouget, Caramel Peanut Butter, Caramel Pecan bar**
1-2 g Net Carbs per bar
  Contains trans fats.

Pure De-lite Dark Chocolate Bar (Phases 2-4)
0 g Net Carbs per bar

Pure De-lite Milk Chocolate Bar (Phases 2-4)
3 g Net Carbs per bar

Pure De-lite White Chocolate Bar (Phases 2-4)
3 g Net Carbs per bar

Pure De-lite Gummy Zoo Animals (Phases 1-4)
0 g Net Carbs per serving

Pure De-lite Mint Pattie (Phases 2-4)
0 g Net Carbs per bar

⚠ **Pure De-lite Peanut Butter Cups**
2 g Net Carbs per piece
  Contains trans fats.

Pure De-lite Truffle Bars, most flavors (Phases 2-4)
2 g Net Carbs per bar

NUTRITION BARS

  See page 250.

➤ FLOUR AND BAKE MIXES ◄

Like their mainstream counterparts, nearly all natural foods store brands of flours and bake mixes are very high in carbs; you will want to use them only in small quantities and mostly in the later phases of Atkins. Although you may not think their Net Carb counts are vastly different, the higher fiber in multigrain mixes for breads, muffins, pancakes and waffles and so on, makes them much more nutritious choices than their bleached white flour counterparts, as are the myriad varieties of whole-grain flours. Seek out flours made from soy, brown rice, oats, rye, spelt, and kamut. Look for Atkins Quick Quisine Bake Mixes and other controlled-carb mixes for foods like breads, muffins, pie crusts, pancakes, and waffles.

FLOUR

Atkins Quick Quisine Bake Mix (Phases 1-4)
3 g Net Carbs per ¼ cup dry mix

Arrowhead Mills Buckwheat Flour (Phases 3 & 4)
18 g Net Carbs per ¼ cup

**Arrowhead Mills Whole Grain Oat Flour
(Phases 3 & 4)**
18 g Net Carbs per ⅓ cup

Arrowhead Mills Whole Grain Soy Flour (Phases 1-4)
4 g Net Carbs per ¼ cup

Almond Meal/Flour (Phases 2-4)
3 g Net Carbs per ¼ cup

Barley Flour (Phases 3 & 4)
15 g Net Carbs per ¼ cup

Flaxseed Meal (Phases 1-4)
0 g Net Carbs per 2 tablespoons

Soy Flour (Phases 1-4)
5 g Net Carbs per ¼ cup

Soy Powder (Phases 1-4)
3.5 g Net Carbs per ¼ cup

Vital Wheat Gluten (Phases 2-4)
6 g Net Carbs per ¼ cup

BAKE MIXES

Atkins Quick Quisine Cookie Mixes, Chocolate Chip, Chocolate Chocolate Chip (Phases 2-4)
6 g Net Carbs per 2 cookies

Atkins Quick Quisine Deluxe Fudge Brownie Mix (Phases 2-4)
9 g Net Carbs per brownie

Atkins Quick Quisine Muffin & Bread Mixes, Blueberry, Corn, Lemon Poppy (Phases 1-4)
3 g Net Carbs per serving

Atkins Quick Quisine Muffin & Bread Mixes, Orange Cranberry, Banana Nut (Phases 1-4)
2 g Net Carbs per serving

Atkins Quick Quisine Muffin & Bread Mixes, Chocolate Chocolate Chip (Phases 2-4)
6 g Net Carbs per serving

Atkins Quick Quisine Pancake & Waffle Mixes (Phases 1-4)
3 g Net Carbs per 1/4 cup dry mix

Atkins Quick Quisine Deluxe Buttermilk Pancake Mix (Phases 2-4)
8 g Net Carbs per ⅓ cup dry mix

FYI **Carborite Bread Mix (Phases 2-4)**
4 g Net Carbs per ¼-inch slice
  Contains flour.

FYI **Carborite Low Carb Pancake Mix (Phases 2-4)**
5 g Net Carbs per 35 grams dry mix
  Contains flour.

Carborite Zero Carb Bake Mix, Vanilla (Phases 1-4)
0 g Net Carbs per 28 grams dry mix

CarbSense Bread Mix, Harvest Wheat (Phases 1-4)
3 g Net Carbs per slice

CarbSense Muffin Mix, Honey Bran (Phases 1-4)
3 g Net Carb per 2 muffins

CarbSense Pancake & Waffle Mix, Buttermilk or Buckwheat (Phases 2-4)
4 g Net Carbs per ½ cup dry mix

CarbSense Pizza Crust Mix, Garlic & Herb (Phases 1-4)
3 g Net Carbs per slice

CarbSense Zero Carb Baking Mix (Phases 1-4)
0 g Net Carbs per ½ cup dry mix

CarbSense MiniCarb Bread Mix, Country White (Phases 1-4)
3 g Net Carbs per slice

CarbSense MiniCarb Buttery Biscuit Mix (Phases 1-4)
0 g Net Carbs per biscuit

CarbSense MiniCarb Cake Mix, Carrot, Chocolate
(Phases 2-4)
4 g Net Carbs per ⅓ cup dry mix

CarbSense MiniCarb Chocolate Brownie Mix
(Phases 2-4)
2 g Net Carbs per brownie

CarbSense MiniCarb Cookie Mix, Snickerdoodle,
Lemon Burst (Phases 2-4)
2 g Net Carbs per cookie

CarbSense MiniCarb Muffin Mix, Apple Cinnamon
(Phases 1-4)
3 g Net Carbs per muffin

CarbSense MiniCarb Muffin Mix, Sweet Corn
(Phases 1-4)
2 g Net Carbs per muffin

CarbSense MiniCarb Pancake Mix, Apple Cinnamon
(Phases 1-4)
1 g Net Carbs per ½ cup dry mix (about 2 pancakes)

CarbSense MiniCarb Pie Crust Mix (Phases 1-4)
1 g Net Carbs per slice

CarbSense MiniCarb Pizza Crust Mix, Parmesan Herb
(Phases 1-4)
3 g Net Carbs per slice

CarbSense MiniCarb Zero Carb Baking Mix (Phases 1-4)
0 g Net Carbs per ½ cup dry mix

Keto Bread Machine Mix, Banana, Pumpernickel, Rye
(Phases 2-4)
2 g Net Carbs per slice

Keto Bread Machine Mix, Cinnamon Raisin (Phases 2-4)
3 g Net Carbs per slice

Keto Bread Machine Mix, French Loaf, Sourdough Rye, Golden Original (Phases 1-4)
2 g Net Carbs per slice

Keto Chocolate Chip Cookie Mix (Phases 2-4)
1 g Net Carbs per cookie

Keto Chocolate Cookie and Brownie Mix (Phases 2-4)
1 g Net Carbs per 2 cookies or 1 brownie

Keto Muffin and Pancake Mix, Golden Original (Phases 1-4)
3 g Net Carbs per 3 pancakes or 2 muffins

Keto Oatmeal Raisin Cookie Mix (Phases 2-4)
1 g Net Carbs per 2 cookies

Keto Pizza Dough (Phases 1-4)
2 g Net Carbs per slice

Keto Pudding, French Vanilla, Chocolate, Banana (Phases 2-4)
1 g Net Carbs per ½ scoop mix

Ketogenics Bread Mixes, most varieties (Phases 1-4)
2 g Net Carbs per slice

Ketogenics Low Carb Muffin Mix, Apple Cinnamon Bran (Phases 1-4)
2 g Net Carbs per muffin

Ketogenics Low Carb Muffin Mix, Chocolate Chip (Phases 1-4)
1 g Net Carbs per muffin

Ketogenics Low Carb Muffin Mix, Wild Blueberry (Phases 1-4)
2 g Net Carbs per muffin

Ketogenics Pancake Mix (Phases 1-4)
5 g Net Carbs per ⅔ cup dry mix

SOY FLOUR VS. SOY POWDER

Wondering about the difference between soy flour and soy powder, and how to use them? Speculate no more. Soy powder is finely ground cooked soybeans. It's used for both baking and making soymilk. Soy flour, used for baking only, is made by grinding whole, uncooked soybeans into flour, in the same way that wheat kernels are ground into flour. Soy flour often contains hull material and is coarser.

➤ GRAINS, BEANS, AND LEGUMES ◄

GRAINS

Once you're approaching the Pre-Maintenance phase of Atkins, you can enjoy the large variety of nutritious whole grains available in your natural foods stores. Unlike refined grains, whole grains—which retain their nutrient-packed bran and germ—are rich in vitamin E, protein, B vitamins, minerals and fiber. Most grains can be prepared in the same way that you cook rice or oatmeal, though they may require longer cooking times. They are done when they're just slightly chewy.

Amaranth (Phases 3 & 4)
50 g Net Carbs per ½ cup cooked

Barley (Phases 3 & 4)
52 g Net Carbs per ½ cup raw

Barley Flakes, rolled (Phases 3 & 4)
23 g Net Carbs per ⅓ cup raw

Barley, hulled (whole-grain) (Phases 3 & 4)
13 Net Carbs per ½ cup cooked

Bob's Red Mill Barley, whole and hull-less (Phases 3 & 4)
26 g Net Carbs per ¼ cup raw

Bob's Red Mill Barley-Rolled Flakes (Phases 3 & 4)
15 g Net Carbs per ¼ cup raw

Bob's Red Mill Flaxseed Meal (Phases 1-4)
0 g Net Carbs per 2 tablespoons raw

Bob's Red Mill Spelt Berries (Phases 3 & 4)
27 g Net Carbs per ¼ cup raw

Bob's Red Mill Spelt Flakes, rolled (Phases 3 & 4)
42 g Net Carbs per ½ cup raw

Bob's Red Mill Triticale Berries (Phases 3 & 4)
25 g Net Carbs per ¼ cup raw

Bob's Red Mill Triticale, rolled flakes (Phases 3 & 4)
18 g Net Carbs per ¼ cup raw

Buckwheat (Phases 3 & 4)
9 g Net Carbs per ½ cup cooked

Bulgur Wheat (Phases 3 & 4)
13 g Net Carbs per ½ cup cooked

Cracked Wheat (Phases 3 & 4)
15 g Net Carbs per ½ cup cooked

Kamut (Phases 3 & 4)
26 g Net Carbs per ½ cup cooked

Millet, whole (Phases 3 & 4)
26 g Net Carbs per ½ cup cooked

Oat Bran (Phases 3 & 4)
19 g Net Carbs per ⅓ cup cooked

Quinoa (Phases 3 & 4)
54 g Net Carbs per ½ cup cooked

Rye Flakes (Phases 3 & 4)
14 g Net Carbs per ½ cup cooked

Teff (Phases 3 & 4)
20 g Net Carbs per ½ cup cooked

Wheat Bran (Phases 1-4)
2 g Net Carbs per 2 tablespoons raw

Wheat Flakes (Phases 3 & 4)
14 g Net Carbs per ½ cup cooked

Wheat Germ, untoasted (Phases 2-4)
3 g Net Carbs per 2 tablespoons

Winter Wheat Berries (Phases 3 & 4)
14 g Net Carbs per ½ cup cooked

BEANS AND LEGUMES

A natural foods store is likely to carry a greater variety of beans and legumes than a mainstream grocery store, including heirloom beans. (See pages 41, 210 and 235 for more on beans.) Beans are an excellent source of digestible and nondigestible fiber and provide generous amounts of protein, but they vary quite a bit in carb counts.

Adzuki Beans (Phases 3 & 4)
20 g Net Carbs per ½ cup cooked

Anasazi Beans (Phases 3 & 4)
13 g Net Carbs per ½ cup cooked
Anasazis look somewhat like red kidney beans with white splotches. They cook somewhat faster than other beans.

Appaloosa Beans (Phases 3 & 4)
9 g Net Carbs per ¼ cup cooked
White with reddish-orange spots, Appaloosas can be used in lieu of pinto beans in most recipes.

Mung Beans (Phases 3 & 4)
14 g Net Carbs per ½ cup cooked
Most commonly encountered as sprouts or ground and formed into bean threads (also called cellophane noodles and common in Chinese cookery), dried mung beans have an olive skin and yellow flesh.

Soybeans, beige or black (Phases 3 & 4)
4 g Net Carbs per ½ cup cooked

Soybeans, green (Phases 3 & 4)
6 g Net Carbs per ½ cup cooked

Trout Beans (Phases 3 & 4)
10 g Net Carbs per ¼ cup cooked

Sometimes called Jacob's Cattle beans or coach beans, these are white beans with maroon spots. Use them in place of pinto or kidney beans in soups.

➤ SOY FOODS AND MEAT ALTERNATIVES ◄

Tofu and other soy foods can be a valuable addition to your eating plan because of their purported health benefits, including reducing the risk of cardiovascular disease and protecting against osteoporosis, along with their relatively low carb content. Plus, the wide variety of products available these days means there's a substitute for practically anything typically made with meat. You can now have your tofu or faux hamburger marinated, baked or hickory smoked—and in flavors such as barbecue, Tex-Mex and ginger teriyaki (though you may find some flavored products to be significantly higher in Net Carbs or high in sugar and other unacceptable ingredients so read labels carefully).

Also, if you haven't been a fan of veggie burgers in the past, it's time to try one again—meat analogs have improved significantly in flavor and texture.

TOFU, SEITAN, AND TEMPEH

Whether you choose soft, silken, firm, or extra firm, tofu supplies 2–3 grams of Net Carbs, ½–2 grams of fiber, and 10–11 grams of protein per ½ cup. Tofu's other nutritional highlights: phytochemicals called isoflavones (see "Phytochemicals" on page 35), as well as calcium, iron, selenium, and folate.

Seitan is wheat gluten cooked in soy sauce. It is firm and chewy, like meat, and very high in protein—a ⅓-cup serving supplies 0–2 grams of fiber and 18–23 grams of protein. You can buy it refrigerated, frozen, in jars, or as a packaged dry mix. Seitan can be kept frozen for up to six months. Seitan, too, is relatively low in carbs.

Tempeh originated in Indonesia. It is a tender, chewy cake made of soybeans that have been fermented with a grain, usually rice or millet. Unlike tofu and seitan, tempeh is almost always cooked before it is eaten, although it can be eaten raw when it's very fresh. Tempeh is a good source of minerals and vitamin B_6. Carb counts vary among brands and flavors. (See page 51 for tofu and seitan.) Because tempeh often contains rice, it may not be appropriate until the later phases of Atkins. If you're a vegetarian following Atkins, you may consider introducing it earlier.

⚠️ **Lightlife Organic Seitan, Barbecue**
9 g Net Carbs per 3 ounces
   Contains added sugars.

Lightlife Organic Seitan, Teriyaki (Phases 2-4)
8 g Net Carbs per 3 ounces

Lightlife Organic Tempeh, Wild Rice (Phases 2-4)
4 g Net Carbs per 4 ounces

Lightlife Organic Tempeh, Garden Veggie (Phases 3 & 4)
13 g Net Carbs per 4 ounces

Lightlife Organic Tempeh, Soy (Phases 2-4)
4 g Net Carbs per 4 ounces

Lightlife Organic Tempeh, 3-Grain (Phases 3 & 4)
13 g Net Carbs per 4 ounces

Turtle Island Foods 5-Grain Tempeh (Phases 3 & 4)
14 g Net Carbs per 3 ounces

Turtle Island Foods Edamame Veggie Tempeh (Phases 3 & 4)
14 g Net Carbs per 3 ounces

Turtle Island Foods Indonesian Tempeh (Phases 3 & 4)
14 g Net Carbs per 3 ounces

Turtle Island Foods Soy Tempeh (Phases 3 & 4)
14 g Net Carbs per 3 ounces

White Wave Baked Tofu, Garlic Herb Italian, Roma Tomato Basil, Zesty Lemon Pepper (Phases 1-4)
0 g Net Carbs per piece

White Wave Baked Tofu, Thai Style (Phase 1-4)
0 g Net Carbs per piece

White Wave 5-Grain Tempeh (Phases 3 & 4)
9 g Net Carbs per ⅓ block

White Wave Original Soy Tempeh (Phases 1-4)
4 g Net Carbs per ⅓ block

White Wave Sea Veggie Tempeh (Phases 1-4)
2 g Net Carbs per ⅓ block

White Wave Seitan, Traditional, Chicken Style (Phases 1-4)
2 g Net Carbs per serving

White Wave Soy Rice Tempeh (Phases 3 & 4)
12 g Net Carbs per ⅓ block

White Wave Tofu, extra firm (Phases 1-4)
2 g Net Carbs per ¼ block

White Wave Tofu, soft (Phases 1-4)
2 g Net Carbs per ⅕ block

MEAT ALTERNATIVES

Whether you're looking for a meat alternative for your backyard barbecue or a more formal feast, you'll find something that fills the bill in your natural foods store. The formulations vary dramatically and so do the flavor, texture, and nutrients. Very low carb counts usually indicate the maker has used a soy protein concentrate or isolate as its primary ingredient. When counts are higher, there are likely to be more beans, vegetables, such as potatoes, or rice at the top of the ingredients list. Quorn products are made with mycoprotein, a fungi and relative of mushrooms, truffles, and morels.

Be aware that a low carb count doesn't necessarily mean a product is okay for all phases—moderate portions of brown rice and potatoes can be introduced in Pre-Maintenance and Lifetime Maintenance.

⚠ Amy's All-American Burger
12 g Net Carbs per patty
  Contains added sugars.

Amy's California Burger (Phases 3 & 4)
14 g Net Carbs per patty

Amy's Chicago Burger (Phases 3 & 4)
17 g Net Carbs per patty

⚠ Amy's Texas Burger
11 g Net Carbs per patty
  Contains added sugars.

Health Is Wealth Buffalo "Wings" (Phases 2-4)
8 g Net Carbs per 3 nuggets

Health Is Wealth Chicken-Free Nuggets (Phases 2-4)
9 g Net Carbs per 3 nuggets

Health Is Wealth Chicken-Free Patties (Phases 3 & 4)
13 g Net Carbs per patty

Lightlife Gimme Lean Ground Beef Style Ground Meat (Phases 1-4)
2 g Net Carbs per 2 ounces

▲ Lightlife Gimme Lean Sausage Style Ground Meat
2 g Net Carbs per 2 ounces
  Contains added sugars.

Lightlife Light Burgers (Phases 1-4)
6 g Net Carbs per patty

Lightlife Organic Tempeh Grilles, Lemon (Phases 2-4)
11 g Net Carbs per patty

Lightlife Organic Tempeh Grilles, Tamari (Phases 2-4)
9 g Net Carbs per patty

▲ Lightlife Organic Tempeh, Fakin' Bacon Strips
5 g Net Carbs per 3 slices
  Contains added sugars.

Nate's Chicken Style Nuggets (Phases 1-4)
2 g Net Carbs per 3 nuggets

Natural Touch Nine-Bean Loaf (Phases 3 & 4)
11 g Net Carbs per slice

Natural Touch Vegetarian Tuno (Phases 1-4)
1 g Net Carbs per ⅓ cup

▲ Quorn Naked Cutlets
3 g Net Carbs per cutlet
  Contains added sugars.

⚠ Quorn Chicken-Style Patties
9 g Net Carbs per patty
Contains added sugars.

⚠ Smart Bacon
2 g Net Carbs per 2 slices
Contains added sugars.

⚠ Smart Cutlets, Seasoned Chick'n
7 g Net Carbs per cutlet
Contains added sugars.

⚠ Smart Deli, Country Ham Style
4 g Net Carbs per 4 slices
Contains added sugars.

⚠ Smart Deli, Old World Bologna Style
2 g Net Carbs per 4 slices
Contains added sugars.

⚠ Smart Deli, Roast Turkey Style
3 g Net Carbs per 4 slices
Contains added sugars.

Smart Dogs Grill Ready Brats (Phases 1-4)
4 g Net Carbs per link

Smart Dogs Tofu Pups (Phases 1-4)
2 g Net Carbs per 3 slices

⚠ Smart Ground Original Ground Meat
2 g Net Carbs per ⅓ cup
Contains added sugars.

⚠ **Smart Ground Taco & Burrito Ground Meat**
4 g Net Carbs per ⅓ cup
  Contains added sugars.

⚠ **Smart Links, Country Breakfast Style**
4 g Net Carbs per 2 links
  Contains added sugars.

FYI **Smart Links, Old World Italian Style (Phases 2–4)**
5 g Net Carbs per link
  Contains potato starch.

⚠ **Smart Menu Chick'n Nuggets**
14 Net Carbs per 4 nuggets
  Contains added sugars.

Smart Menu Chick'n Strips (Phases 1–4)
3 g Net Carbs per 3 ounces

Smart Menu Steak-Style Strips (Phases 1–4)
3 g Net Carbs per 3 ounces

⚠ **Smart Cutlets, Salisbury Steak Style**
5 g Net Carbs per cutlet
  Contains added sugars.

Tofurky Beerbrats (Phases 2–4)
6 g Net Carbs per 3.5 ounces

**Tofurky Deli Slices, Original, Peppered, Hickory
Smoked (Phases 3 & 4)**
15 g Net Carbs per 3 slices

⚠ **Tofurky Jurky, Original, Ginger Teriyaki, Peppered**
8 g Net Carbs per 4 pieces
  Contains added sugars.

Tofurky Kielbasa (Phases 2-4)
6 g Net Carbs per 3.5 ounces

Tofurky Roast, Whole Turkey (Phases 2-4)
8 g Net Carbs per 4 ounces

Tofurky Sweet Italian Sausage (Phases 2-4)
9 g Net Carbs per 3.5 ounces

Turtle Island Foods Super Burgers, Original, Smoked (Phases 3 & 4)
14 g Net Carbs per patty

Turtle Island Foods Super Burgers, Tex Mex (Phases 3 & 4)
11 g Net Carbs per patty

⚠️ **Veat Chick'n Free Nuggets**
3 g Net Carbs per 70-gram serving
  Contains added sugars.

⚠️ **Veat Gourmet Bites**
7 g Net Carbs per 70-gram serving
  Contains added sugars.

⚠️ **Veat Vegetarian Breast**
5 g Net Carbs per 50-gram serving
  Contains added sugars.

➤ MISCELLANEOUS MIXES AND BOXED MEALS ◄

Most of the meat analogs, or substitutes, are in the refrigerator or freezer case, but you'll find mixes for soup, chili, tacos, and the like in the dry foods aisles as well.

Fantastic Foods Instant Refried Beans (Phases 3 & 4)
15 g Net Carbs per ¼ cup dry mix

Fantastic Foods Falafel (Phases 3 & 4)
16 g Net Carbs per ¼ cup dry mix

Fantastic Foods Hummus Original, Spinach, Parmesan (Phases 3 & 4)
10 g Net Carbs per 2 tablespoons dry mix

⚠ **Fantastic Foods Sloppy Joe Mix**
8 g Net Carbs per ¼ cup dry mix
  Contains added sugars.

Fantastic Foods Tabouli Mix (Phases 3 & 4)
11 g Net Carbs per 2 tablespoons dry mix

Fantastic Foods Tofu Burger Mix (Phases 3 & 4)
12 g Net Carbs per 3 tablespoons dry mix

⚠ **Fantastic Foods Taco Filling**
6 g Net Carbs per ¼ cup dry mix
  Contains added sugars.

Fantastic Foods Tofu Scrambler (Phases 2-4)
6 g Net Carbs per tablespoon dry mix

⚠ **Fantastic Foods Vegetarian Chili**
13 g Net Carbs per ¼ cup dry mix
  Contains added sugars.

Soy Protein Mix, most brands (Phases 1-4)
1 g Net Carbs per 3 tablespoons dry mix

Textured Vegetable Protein, most brands (Phases 1-4)
3 g Net Carbs per dry ounce

➤ BEVERAGES ◄

SOYMILK

The problem with soymilk and other nondairy beverages is that most are overly sweetened with unacceptable ingredients, therefore upping the carb count. Look for unsweetened soymilk or soymilk sweetened with sucralose; these have fewer than 5 grams of Net Carbs per serving.

If you like flavored soymilk, look for WestSoy's Soy Slender, which has 1 gram of Net Carbs. Other cow's milk substitutes, such as kefir or creamy beverages made from oat, rice, almond and other nuts and grains, all have high carb counts, often from sweeteners. (See also pages 125 and 273.) Goat's milk is permitted after Induction.

Edensoy, unsweetened (Phases 1-4)
3 g Net Carbs per cup

Silk Organic, unsweetened (Phases 2-4)
4 g Net Carbs per cup

Vitasoy Original, unsweetened (Phases 2-4)
5 g Net Carbs per cup

WestSoy Organic, unsweetened (Phases 1-4)
1 g Net Carbs per cup

WestSoy Soy Slender, Vanilla, Chocolate, Cappuccino (Phases 1-4)
1 g Net Carbs per cup

DRINK MIXES AND SHAKES

Atkins Advantage Ready-to-Drink Shakes, Creamy Vanilla, Chocolate Delight (Phases 1-4)
1 g Net Carbs per can

Atkins Advantage Ready-to-Drink Shakes, Chocolate Royale, Café au Lait, Strawberry Supreme (Phases 1-4)
2 g Net Carbs per can

Atkins Advantage Spoon-Stirrable Shake Mixes, all flavors (Phases 1-4)
3 g Net Carbs per 2 scoops

Atkins Morning Start Drink Mixes, all flavors (Phases 1-4)
0 g Net Carbs per 8 ounces

Carborite At Last! Ready to Drink Chocolate Shake (Phases 1-4)
2 g Net Carbs per can

Carborite At Last! Ready to Drink Vanilla Shake (Phases 1-4)
1 g Net Carbs per can

Carborite Shake Mix, most flavors (Phases 1-4)
3 g Net Carbs per serving

Doctor's CarbRite Diet Smoothie, most flavors (Phases 1-4)
2 g Net Carbs per scoop

Doctor's CarbRite Diet Soy Creations, most flavors (Phases 1-4)
0 g Net Carbs per scoop

Keto Carb Kooler Mix, Cranberry, Grape (Phases 1-4)
0 g Net Carbs per teaspoon

Keto Chocolate Milk (Phases 1-4)
2 g Net Carbs per scoop

Keto Hot Cocoa (Phases 1-4)
2 g Net Carbs per scoop

Keto Milk (Phases 1-4)
1 g Net Carbs per scoop

Keto Ready-to-Drink Shakes, Chocolate (Phases 1-4)
2 g Net Carbs per container

**Keto Ready-to-Drink Shakes, Vanilla
(Phases 1-4)**
1 g Net Carbs per container

Keto Shakes, most flavors (Phases 1-4)
1 g Net Carbs per 2 scoops

Keto Soy Shake, most flavors (Phases 1-4)
3 g Net Carbs per 2 scoops

Low Carb Creations Sippers, most flavors (Phases 1-4)
1 g Net Carbs per serving

➤ NUT AND SEED BUTTERS ◄

If you're looking to break out of the peanut butter rut (most commercial peanut butter brands are loaded with sugar and hydrogenated oil), you'll find an array of delightful nut and seed butters in natural foods stores. These butters are rich in protein, fiber and essential fatty acids—each with a slightly different mix of nutrients. Their carb counts vary, but all have less than 10 grams of Net Carbs per 2 tablespoons. You'll notice these nut butters look different from commercial peanut butter. Because they are not emulsified with hydrogenated oils, the oil sits on top of the butter—stir them thoroughly before using.

Arrowhead Mills Almond Butter, crunchy (Phases 2-4)
5 g Net Carbs per 2 tablespoons

Arrowhead Mills Cashew Butter, crunchy (Phases 2-4)
7 g Net Carbs per 2 tablespoons

Arrowhead Mills Sesame Tahini (Phases 2-4)
3 g Net Carbs per 2 tablespoons

Beanit Butter (Phases 2-4)
1 g Net Carbs per 2 tablespoons

I.M. Healthy Low Carb Soy Nut Butter, creamy, chunky (Phases 2-4)
1 g Net Carbs per 2 tablespoons

Marantha Cashew Macadamia Butter (Phases 2-4)
6 g Net Carbs per 2 tablespoons

Marantha Macadamia Nut Butter (Phases 2-4)
2 g Net Carbs per 2 tablespoons

Marantha Organic Almond Butter, crunchy (Phases 2-4)
3 g Net Carbs per 2 tablespoons

Marantha Organic Cashew Butter (Phases 2-4)
9 g Net Carbs per 2 tablespoons

Marantha Organic Raw Tahini, no salt (Phases 2-4)
6 g Net Carbs per 2 tablespoons

Marantha Organic Roasted Tahini, no salt (Phases 2-4)
8 g Net Carbs per 2 tablespoons

Marantha Raw Almond Butter, creamy (Phases 2-4)
2 g Net Carbs per 2 tablespoons

Natural Touch Roasted Soy Butter (Phases 2-4)
9 g Net Carbs per 2 tablespoons

Sunny Nut Butter Sunflower Seed Butter (Phases 2-4)
1 g Net Carbs per 2 tablespoons

Tohum Sesame Tahini (Phases 2-4)
3 g Net Carbs per 2 tablespoons

Woodstock Farms Cashew Butter, unsalted (Phases 2-4)
9 g Net Carbs per 2 tablespoons

Woodstock Farms Organic Almond Butter, unsalted (Phases 2-4)
3 g Net Carbs per 2 tablespoons

Woodstock Farms Sesame Tahini (Phases 2-4)
0 g Net Carbs per 2 tablespoons

➤ PASTAS AND PASTA MIXES ◄

Alternatives to regular white flour pasta include pastas made from brown rice, quinoa, kamut, soy and spelt. Unfortunately, while these kinds of grains make pasta far more healthful in terms of nutrients and fiber (see "Grains" on pages 232 and 336), they don't bring the carb count down much. Regular pasta averages about 42–43 grams of Net Carbs per cup cooked, and these varieties range from about 35–45 grams. Kamut is the lowest, at 27 grams of Net Carbs per cup cooked, so if you eat only a half-cup, it's just 13.5 grams of Net Carbs. Soy pastas, however, can be very low in carbs. There are also several brands of controlled-carb pastas to choose from, including Atkins Quick Quisine Pasta Cuts. (Remember, you'll need to add in carbs for any pasta sauce.)

Atkins Quick Quisine Pasta Cuts, Penne, Rotini, Spaghetti (Phases 2-4)
5 g Net Carbs per 2 ounces dry

Atkins Quick Quisine Pasta Sides, Fettuccine Alfredo, Pesto Cream (Phases 2-4)
7 g Net Carbs per serving

Atkins Quick Quisine Pasta Sides, Elbows & Cheese (Phases 2-4)
8 g Net Carbs per serving

Ancient Harvest Quinoa Pasta (Phases 3 & 4)
32.5 g Net Carbs per 2 ounces dry

CarbSense Aramana Pasta Meal Mix, Creamy Chicken Alfredo, Mild Mexican Chicken, Cheddar Cheeseburger (Phases 2-4)
6 g Net Carbs per ⅕ box

Darielle Pasta Elbows (Phases 2-4)
10 g Net Carbs per ¾ cup dry

Darielle Pasta Fusilli (Phases 2-4)
10 g Net Carbs per ¾ cup dry

Darielle Pasta Mezze Penne (Phases 2-4)
10 g Net Carbs per ¾ cup dry

DeBoles Carb Fit Pasta, Elbows, Spaghetti, Rotini (Phases 2-4)
9 g Net Carbs per 2-ounce serving

DeBoles Carb Fit Pasta, Penne (Phases 2-4)
8 g Net Carbs per ½ cup

Due Amici Pasta Lite Low Carb Pasta, Rigatoni, Penne Rigate (Phases 2-4)
3 g Net Carbs per ¾ cup

Keto Pasta, Elbows (Phases 2-4)
5 g Net Carbs per ⅓ cup dry

Keto High-Protein Macaroni and Cheese Dinner (Phases 2-4)
5 g Net Carbs per 1⅔ ounces dry

Keto High-Protein Shells (Phases 2-4)
5 g Net Carbs per ¼ cup dry

Keto High-Protein Spaghetti (Phases 2-4)
5 g Net Carbs per 1.3 ounces dry

Pastalia Heart-Healthy Low-Carb Pasta, Tomato Basil (Phases 2-4)
7 g Net Carbs per 2 ounces dry

Vitaspelt Whole Grain Spelt Pasta (Phases 3 & 4)
35 g Net Carbs per 2 ounces dry

➤ SALAD DRESSINGS ◄

Natural brands of dressings can add zip to your greens, and some contain expeller-pressed oils and less sugar than mainstream brands. However, most still fall short when it comes to fitting into a healthy, controlled-carb lifestyle. Be on the lookout for ingredients like cane sugar and honey.

Atkins Quick Quisine Salad Dressings, "Sweet As Honey" Mustard, Lemon Poppyseed, Country French, Ranch (Phases 1-4)
1 g Net Carbs per 2 tablespoons

Steel's Gourmet Salad Dressing, Honey Mustard (Phases 1-4)
0 g Net Carbs per tablespoon

Steel's Gourmet Salad Dressing, Sweet Ginger Lime (Phases 1-4)
1 g Net Carbs per tablespoon

Sweet William Shallot Vinaigrette (Phases 1-4)
0 Net Carbs per tablespoon

➤ SAUCES, CONDIMENTS, ◄ AND MARINADES

From sweet-tooth-tempting dessert toppings to reduced-carb bread spreads to main meal dips and sauces, the items in this category can help enhance your favorite entrees and snacks. But be careful: The products in these categories should be examined carefully, since they often contain hidden sugars. While the natural brands may use honey and fruit juices instead of sugar and corn syrup, the basic recipes are the same as those used for major brands, and the carb counts aren't significantly different. Mustard, mayonnaise, and hot sauces contain negligible amounts of carbs. Watch your dipping and grilling sauces, too.

Atkins Quick Quisine Sauces, Ketch-a-Tomato, Barbeque, Steak and Teriyaki (Phases 1-4)
1 g Net Carbs per tablespoon

Colac Dessert Toppings (Phases 2-4)
1 g Net Carbs per tablespoon

Colac Jellies, most flavors (Phases 2-4)
1 g Net Carbs per tablespoon

⚠️ **Eden Ponzu Sauce**
1 g Net Carbs per tablespoon
  Contains added sugars.

Fifty-50 Fruit Spreads, Grape, Strawberry, Apple, Orange Marmalade and others (Phases 2-4)
4 g Net Carbs per tablespoon

Fifty-50 Syrups, Chocolate (Phases 2-4)
7 g Net Carbs per 2 tablespoons

Jok 'N' Al Apple Sauce (Phases 3 & 4)
1 g Net Carbs per tablespoon

⚠️ **Jok 'N' Al Cranberry Sauce**
2 g Net Carbs per tablespoon
  Contains added sugars.

Keto Butta (Phases 1-4)
0 g Net Carbs per teaspoon

⚠️ **Keto Fruit Spreads, all flavors**
2 g Net Carbs per tablespoon
  Contains added sugars.

Keto Ketchup (Phases 1-4)
1 g Net Carbs per tablespoon

Keto Pancake Syrup (Phases 1-4)
1 g Net Carbs per ¼ cup

La Nouba Cocoa Spread (Phases 2-4)
4 g Net Carbs per tablespoon

La Nouba Sugar-Free Fruit Spreads, most flavors (Phases 2-4)
8 g Net Carbs per tablespoon

Santa Cruz Organic Apple Apricot Sauce (Phases 3 & 4)
11 g Net Carbs per ½ cup

**Santa Cruz Organic Apple Blackberry Sauce
(Phases 3 & 4)**
11 g Net Carbs per ½ cup

**Santa Cruz Organic Apple Cinnamon Sauce
(Phases 3 & 4)**
17 g Net Carbs per ½ cup

Santa Cruz Organic Apple Sauce (Phases 3 & 4)
13 g Net Carbs per ½ cup

**Santa Cruz Organic Apple Strawberry Sauce
(Phases 3 & 4)**
11 g Net Carbs per ½ cup

Steel's Breakfast Syrup, Country Maple (Phases 1-4)
0 g Net Carbs per 3 tablespoons

Steel's Cocktail Sauce with Dill and Lemon (Phases 1-4)
1 g Net Carbs per 4 tablespoons

**Steel's Dessert Sauce, Caramel, Chocolate Fudge,
Peanut Butter Fudge (Phases 2-4)**
3 g Net Carbs per 2 tablespoons

**Steel's Jam, Apricot, Champagne Peach, Raspberry,
Sour Cherry, Wild Blueberry, Strawberry (Phases 2-4)**
2 g Net Carbs per tablespoon

Steel's Mango Curry Sauce (Phases 2-4)
3 g Net Carbs per tablespoon

Steel's Mango Ginger Chutney (Phases 2-4)
5 g Net Carbs per 5 tablespoons

Steel's Raspberry Jalapeño Sauce (Phases 2-4)
2 g Net Carbs per tablespoon

Steel's Rocky Mountain Barbecue Sauce (Phases 1-4)
2 g Net Carbs per 2 tablespoons

Steel's Rocky Mountain Hoisin Sauce (Phases 1-4)
1 g Net Carbs per 2 tablespoons

Steel's Rocky Mountain Ketchup (Phases 1-4)
0 g Net Carbs per tablespoon

Steel's Rocky Mountain Peanut Sauce (Phases 2-4)
2 g Net Carbs per tablespoon

**Steel's Rocky Mountain Sweet & Sour Sauce
(Phases 1-4)**
2 g Net Carbs per tablespoon

Steel's Spiced Cranberry Sauce (Phases 2-4)
4 g Net Carbs per 5 tablespoons

**Westbrae Naturals Unsweetened Un-Ketchup
(Phases 1-4)**
1 g Net Carbs per tablespoon

➤ SEASONING BLENDS AND BREAD CRUMBS ◄

**A. Vogel Herbamare Organic Herb Seasoning Salt
(Phases 1-4)**
0 g Net Carbs

**A. Vogel Trocomare Organic Spicy Herb Seasoning Salt
(Phases 1-4)**
0 g Net Carbs

Keto Crumbs, Cajun (Phases 2-4)
4 g Net Carbs per ½ cup

Keto Crumbs, Italian and Original (Phases 2-4)
4 g Net Carbs per ¼ cup

➤ SOUPS ◄

In general, dried soup mixes are higher in carbs than are heat-and-serve soups, and broth- or vegetable-based soups are higher in carbs than creamy varieties. You may be surprised, but chicken noodle or chicken and rice soups can be lower in carbs than those chock-full of beans and vegetables. However, avoid those containing noodles made from bleached flour and white rice.

Almost without exception, the soups found in natural foods stores are going to be lower in carbs, added sugars and sodium, and higher in fiber and other nutrients than most major brands in supermarkets. Most natural soups have Net Carb counts between 10 and 15 grams per 1-cup serving. Tomato, bean and split pea soups tend to be higher.

Alpine Aire Instant Low-Carb Soup, Bay Shrimp Bisque, Mushroom & Chicken with Garlic (Phases 2-4)
6 g Net Carbs per container

Alpine Aire Instant Low-Carb Soup, Beefy Vegetable (Phases 2-4)
5 g Net Carbs per container

Alpine Aire Instant Low-Carb Soup, Broccoli & Cheddar, Chicken with Asparagus (Phases 2-4)
4 g Net Carbs per container

Alpine Aire Instant Low-Carb Soup, Chicken Vegetable (Phases 1-4)
3 g Net Carbs per container

Amy's Organic Low Fat Black Bean Vegetable (Phases 3 & 4)
20 g Net Carbs per cup

FYI **Amy's Organic Cream of Mushroom (Phases 3 & 4)**
11 g Net Carbs per ¾ cup
  Contains wheat flour.

Amy's Organic Lentil (Phases 3 & 4)
10 g Net Carbs per cup

Amy's Organic Lentil Vegetable (Phases 3 & 4)
14 g Net Carbs per cup

Amy's Organic Vegetable Broth (Phases 2-4)
7 g Net Carbs per cup

CarbSense MiniCarb Instant Soup Mix, Miso Tofu & Shiitake (Phases 1-4)
4 g Net Carbs per cup

CarbSense MiniCarb Instant Soup Mix, Szechuan Beef (Phases 1-4)
2 g Net Carbs per cup

CarbSense MiniCarb Instant Soup Mix, Thai Coconut Cream (Phases 1-4)
4 g Net Carbs per cup

Fantastic Carb 'Tastic Soup Vegetarian Quick Meals, Asian Ginger Broccoli (Phases 1-4)
3 g Net Carbs per container

Fantastic Carb 'Tastic Soup Vegetarian Quick Meals, Broccoli Cheddar (Phases 2-4)
5 g Net Carbs per container

Fantastic Carb 'Tastic Soup Vegetarian Quick Meals, Shiitake Mushroom, Vegetarian Beef with Barley, Sundried Tomato Basil (Phases 2-4)
6 g Net Carbs per container

⚠️ **Fantastic Carb 'Tastic Soup Vegetarian Quick Meals, Hot and Sour, Vegetarian Mandarin Chicken**
6 g Net Carbs per container
  Contains added sugars.

⚠️ **Fantastic Carb 'Tastic Soup Vegetarian Quick Meals, Vegetarian Chicken Gumbo**
5 g Net Carbs per container
  Contains added sugars.

Shelton's Black Bean and Chicken Soup (Phases 3 & 4)
15 g Net Carbs per cup

Shelton's Chicken Rice Soup (Phases 3 & 4)
12 g Net Carbs per cup

Shelton's Chicken Tortilla Soup (Phases 3 & 4)
12 g Net Carbs per cup

Shelton's Free Range Mild Chicken Chili, Spicy Chicken Chili (Phases 3 & 4)
19 g Net Carbs per cup

SPOTLIGHT ON SEA VEGETABLES

Sea vegetables, more commonly known as seaweed, are nutrient powerhouses and one of the relatively small number of non-animal sources of complete protein. They are also a great source of vitamins—especially A, C, E and the B-group vitamins—and they have a complete set of the minerals required by humans. There's more: Sea vegetables contain a substance that is converted into vitamin D in the body, and they are rich in fiber and extremely low in Net Carbs. Most go by their Japanese names, such as arame, kombu, wakame and hiziki—because they're sold dehydrated, the majority require soaking before cooking. Dulse and nori, however, can be eaten right out of the package. You can add bits of sea vegetables to almost any dish, from soups and salads to grains, vegetables, beans and fish. They will keep for several years when stored in a cool, dry place.

➤ TRAIL MIX ◄

Trail mixes are by no means a low-carb snack. However, they can be a filling and nutritious source of quick energy when you're in the later phases of Atkins, so it's worth seeking out acceptable mixes. For the most part, lower-carb renditions will be simpler combinations consisting mostly of nuts and seeds. That's not to say you won't come across lower-carb mixes with a few chocolate chips tossed in—but steer clear of these, since they likely contain sugar.

Also, avoid mixes with dried fruits and raisins, and any with yogurt-covered nuts or raisins. Instead, look for a mixture of nuts and seeds and unsweetened coconut. Remember, too, you can always create your own trail mix by combining your favorite lower-carb ingredients—go one better by dividing the mix into portioned-controlled individual servings, since it can be all too easy to keep dipping into a bigger bag.

⚠ **GeniSoy Trail Mixes, Happy Trails, Mountain Medley, Tropical Paradise**
14-16 g Net Carbs per ounce
  Contains added sugars.

Kettle Foods Deluxe Mix (Phases 2-4)
4 g Net Carbs per ¼ cup

Kettle Foods Kenai River Mix (Phases 2-4)
4 g Net Carbs per ¼ cup

Kettle Foods Orchard Harvest (Phases 3 & 4)
14 g Net Carbs per ¼ cup

Kettle Foods Raw Hiker's Mix (Phases 3 & 4)
13 g Net Carbs per ¼ cup

Kettle Foods X-Treme Trail Mix (Phases 2-4)
7 g Net Carbs per ¼ cup

Sunridge Farms Cocono Deluxe Mix (Phases 2-4)
9 g Net Carbs per ¼ cup

Sunridge Farms Cranberry Jubilee (Phases 2-4)
8 g Net Carbs per ¼ cup

Sunridge Farms Deluxe Trail Mix (Phases 2-4)
9 g Net Carbs per ¼ cup

Sunridge Farms Hit the Trail Mix (Phases 3 & 4)
10 g Net Carbs per ¼ cup

Sunridge Farms Organic Deluxe Trail Mix (Phases 3 & 4)
11 g Net Carbs per ¼ cup

Sunridge Farms Roasted Tamari Nut Mix (Phases 2-4)
5 g Net Carbs per ¼ cup

Sunridge Farms Tropical Trail Mix (Phases 3 & 4)
10 g Net Carbs per ¼ cup

Woodstock Farms Organic Trail Mix (Phases 3 & 4)
10 g Net Carbs per ¼ cup

➤ YOGURT ◄

Natural foods stores carry yogurts made from the milk of animals other than cows, and these tend to be slightly lower in carbohydrate than supermarket brands. Also, keep an eye out for Atkins-Approved Hood Carb Countdown yogurts, with 3 or 4 grams of Net Carbs per serving (see page 127).

Brown Cow Whole Milk Yogurt, plain (Phases 3 & 4)
12 g Net Carbs per cup

Erivan Acidophilus Yogurt, whole milk (Phases 3 & 4)
11 g Net Carbs per cup

Goat's Milk Yogurt, plain (Phases 3 & 4)
10 g Net Carbs per cup

Sheep's Milk Yogurt, plain (Phases 3 & 4)
8 g Net Carbs per cup

Greek Yogurt, 2% or Fat Free (Phases 3 & 4)
8 g Net Carbs per cup

Yo-Goat Yogurt Drink (Phases 3 & 4)
6 g Net Carbs per cup

➤ FROZEN FOODS ◄

ICE CREAM, FROZEN DESSERT MIXES, AND ICE CREAM SUBSTITUTES

Controlled-carb versions of your favorite ice creams and frozen desserts are being introduced to supermarkets and natural foods stores at an ever-increasing rate. Your best bet is to aim for full-fat products, which are lower in carbs than reduced-fat styles. Atkins Endulge Super Premium Ice Cream products do the Net Carb math for you, but when it comes to other brands, subtract sugar alcohols and glycerine from the grams of total carbohydrates to determine the grams of Net Carbs. And watch out for seemingly healthy soymilk and vegetarian frozen desserts—most contain sugar.

If you have an ice cream maker, making controlled-carb ice cream and frozen dessert mixes is another option.

Atkins Endulge Super Premium Ice Cream Pints, Vanilla, Chocolate, Butter Pecan, Chocolate Peanut Butter Swirl, Chocolate Fudge Brownie, Vanilla Fudge Swirl, Vanilla Swiss Almond, Mint Chocolate Chip (Phases 2-4)
3 g Net Carbs per ½ cup

Atkins Endulge Super Premium Ice Cream Cups, Vanilla, Chocolate, Strawberry, Butter Pecan (Phases 2-4)
4 g Net Carbs per 4-ounce cup

Atkins Endulge Super Premium Ice Cream Bars, Chocolate Fudge (Phases 2-4)
2 g Net Carbs per bar

Atkins Endulge Super Premium Ice Cream Bars, Chocolate Fudge Swirl, Peanut Butter Fudge Swirl, Vanilla Fudge Swirl (Phases 2-4)
3 g Net Carbs per bar

Carborite 4 Soft Serve, both flavors (Phases 1-4)
4 g Net Carbs per ½ cup

Keto Ice Cream Mix, Vanilla, Chocolate, Strawberry, Black Raspberry, Orange and Crème (Phases 2-4)
1 g Net Carbs per ½ cup prepared

Keto Sherbet Mix, Lemon, Orange, Watermelon (Phases 2-4)
2 g Net Carbs per ½ cup prepared

Pure De-lite Premium Ice Cream, Rich Chocolate, Double Chocolate Chunk, Natural Vanilla, Vanilla Chocolate Almond (Phases 2-4)
3 g Net Carbs per serving

RiceDream Non-Dairy Frozen Dessert, Vanilla, Carob (Phases 3 & 4)
22 g Net Carbs per serving

⚠ **SoyDream Non-Dairy Frozen Dessert, French Vanilla**
16 g Net Carbs per serving
  Contains added sugars.

ENTREES AND SIDES

Dr. Praeger's Homestyle Broccoli Pancakes (Phases 2-4)
8 g Net Carbs per pancake

Dr. Praeger's Homestyle Spinach Pancakes (Phases 2-4)
8 g Net Carbs per pancake

Dr. Praeger's Potato Pancakes (Phases 3 & 4)
9 g Net Carbs per pancake

**Dr. Praeger's Veggie Royale Salmon Veggie Burgers
(Phases 2-4)**
10 g Net Carbs per burger

Omega Foods Mahi Mahi Burgers (Phases 1-4)
2 g Net Carbs per patty

Omega Foods Salmon Burgers (Phases 1-4)
3 g Net Carbs per patty

Omega Foods Tuna Burgers (Phases 1-4)
3 g Net Carbs per patty

Shelton's Free Range Turkey Meatballs (Phases 1-4)
6 g Net Carbs per 6 meatballs

POTPIES, SANDWICH POCKETS, AND BUN MEALS

Most potpies, pocket sandwiches and the like boast bleached white flour crusts—and sky high carb counts. Natural foods stores frequently stock items that feature whole-grain crusts and other wholesome ingredients, which can mean they're higher in fiber and other nutrients.

Despite some nutritious, wholesome fillings, most sand-

wich pockets and bun meals have per-serving Net Carb
counts in the 30–40-gram range.

Amy's Organic Shepherd's Pie (Phases 3 & 4)
22 g Net Carbs per pie

Amy's Organic Mexican Tamale Pie (Phases 3 & 4)
23 g Net Carbs per pie

Ian's Beef Shepherd's Pie (Phases 3 & 4)
21 g Net Carbs per 5 ounces

**Shelton's Free Range Whole Wheat Chicken Pie,
Turkey Pie (Phases 3 & 4)**
15 g Net Carbs per 9 ounces

MACARONI AND SOY CHEESE

Unless you find a controlled-carb pasta product, macaroni
and soy cheese will not be much lower in carbs than the
classic versions. Reserve those for the later phases of Atkins
and eat them in moderation.

**Atkins Quick Quisine Pasta Sides, Fettuccine Alfredo,
Pesto Cream (Phases 2-4)**
7 g Net Carbs per cup

**Atkins Quick Quisine Pasta Sides, Elbows & Cheese
(Phases 2-4)**
8 g Net Carbs per cup

FYI Amy's Organic Macaroni and Soy Cheeze
(Phases 3 & 4)
38 g Net Carbs per 9 ounces
Contains wheat flour.

MEXICAN DISHES

Individually packaged frozen burritos are popular items at natural foods stores, but they are not low-carb items. Amy's and Cedarlane burritos have Net Carb gram counts in the 30s and 40s and can be a very occasional option during the later phases of Atkins, if you have a high carb threshold.

Amy's Cheese Enchilada (Phases 3 & 4)
16 g Net Carbs per 4¾ ounces

Cedarlane Cheese Enchiladas (Phases 3 & 4)
17 g Net Carbs per enchilada

Cedarlane Organic Five Layer Mexican Dip (Phases 2-4)
3 g Net Carbs per 2 tablespoons

PIZZAS

Even with whole-grain crusts and soy cheese, frozen pizza is a high-carb choice, with almost all natural brands ranging from 30–40 grams of Net Carbs. Go for controlled-carb renderings or make your own using controlled-carb tortillas or crust mixes.

FYI **Atkins Quick Quisine Pizza, Supreme, Smokehouse, Pepperoni (Phases 2-4)**
11 g Net Carbs per pizza
Contains nitrates.

⚠ Amy's Rice Crust Cheese Pizza
29 g Net Carbs per 4-ounce slice
Contains added sugars.

Darielle Pizza (Phases 2-4)
10 g Net Carbs per ½ pizza

Ian's Natural Foods 4-Cheese Pizza (Phases 2-4)
5 g Net Carbs per slice

Ian's Natural Foods Spinach and 4-Cheese Pizza (Phases 2-4)
4 g Net Carbs per slice

MAKING SENSE OF LABELING

Whether you shop for food at a supermarket, a natural foods store, a warehouse, or a farmer's market, you'll see products bearing a baffling number of labels and acronyms. The good news is that most of these terms are legally defined—that is, the government has developed a set of criteria that foods bearing a label must meet. Here's a quick rundown of what it all means.

ORGANIC

National standards for labeling organic foods began in 2002. Since then, foods produced in accordance with USDA National Organic Program regulations can be labeled organic. Foods containing ingredients produced with pesticides, antibiotics, irradiation or genetic engineering cannot carry any organic label. Within the organic category, here's what you'll find:

- **100% organic:** Products must contain only organically produced ingredients, excluding water and salt.
- **Organic:** Products must consist of at least 95% organically produced ingredients, excluding water and salt.
- **Made with organic [may list up to three ingredients]:** Multi-ingredient products that contain at least 70% organic ingredients can use the phrase "made with organic ingredients."
- **Organic ingredients listed on ingredient panel only:** Multi-ingredient products that contain less than

70% organic ingredients are allowed to list the organic items on the ingredient panel only.

- **Organic meat and poultry:** Animals are fed only organic feed, are given no antibiotics or growth hormones and are taken care of in a humane way, appropriate to their species, and with access to the outdoors.

TRANSITIONAL

To obtain organic certification, a farm has to have been "clean" for three years. Occasionally, you will see products grown on farms that are using organic methods but have not reached their three-year mark yet. Foods from these farms are labeled "transitional." This label is not regulated.

NATURAL

At the national level, the term "natural" is only regulated for meat and poultry products. It means that these animal products are no more than minimally processed and contain no added artificial ingredients. The term is unregulated (except in certain states) for use with other foods, though it generally means that no artificial flavors or colors have been added. It doesn't mean that the product is free of toxic pesticides, fertilizers, sewage sludge, or other undesirable contaminants.

NON-GMO OR NON-GEO

GMO and GEO stand for genetically modified or genetically engineered organisms. When a food is genetically modified or engineered, its genes have been rearranged. There is neither a definitive test yet for all types of food, nor a way to regulate these labeling terms.

RAISED WITHOUT ANTIBIOTICS

Some farmers give their animals prophylactic antibiotics for reasons that range from keeping away bacterial infections to reducing the negative effects of stress and making them retain water so they'll weigh more (and so go for a bigger price). When you see this label, it means the animal was not given any antibiotics. (If an animal gets an infection, it is treated with antibiotics and not given this label.) The effects of animal antibiotics on humans who consume their meat, eggs, or milk are unknown.

RAISED WITHOUT ADDED HORMONES
Some farmers give their animals synthetic hormones to make them grow faster or bigger. The effects of these growth hormones on the humans that consume these animals and their products are unknown.

FREE RANGE, FREE ROAMING, FREE WALKING, CAGE-FREE
These phrases mean the animals are not penned up in cages or small spaces, and are instead allowed to move around and graze in a way that is natural for their species. Depending on the animals, these areas may be indoors.

GLUTEN-FREE
Gluten is a component of grains found in greatest concentrations in wheat, barley, and rye. Gluten causes allergic reactions in certain people (celiac disease is a condition defined by an intolerance to gluten). However, a gluten-free diet may also be beneficial in the treatment of a host of other conditions, ranging from skin conditions to mental illness.

DAIRY-FREE
Dairy-free means a product contains no milk, cheese, butter, cream cheese, cottage cheese, sour cream or ice cream. The most common reason for following a dairy-free diet is an allergy to dairy products, whether it's due to lactose-intolerance or dairy protein. Some people who are extremely lactose-intolerant may also be unable to tolerate other dairy products.

Atkins Food Products

Look for these and other Atkins-brand products at your supermarket and natural foods store.

Breakfast Options
Atkins Morning Start Breakfast Bars
Atkins Morning Start Cereals
Atkins Morning Start Drink Mixes

Meal Replacements
Atkins Advantage Bars
Atkins Advantage Ready-to-Drink Shakes
Atkins Advantage Spoon-Stirrable Shake Mixes

Breads and Baked Goods
Atkins Bakery Dinner Rolls
Atkins Bakery Hot Dog Rolls
Atkins Bakery Ready-to-Eat Muffins
Atkins Bakery Ready-to-Eat Sliced Bagels
Atkins Bakery Ready-to-Eat Sliced Bread
Atkins Bakery Sandwich Rolls
Atkins Bakery Tortillas

Cooking and Baking
Atkins Quick Quisine Bake Mix
Atkins Quick Quisine Chocolate Chip Cookie Mix

Atkins Quick Quisine Deluxe Fudge Brownie Mix
Atkins Quick Quisine Muffin & Bread Mixes
Atkins Quick Quisine Pancake & Waffle Mixes

Entrees and Side Dishes
Atkins Quick Quisine Frozen Individual Pizzas
Atkins Quick Quisine Pasta Cuts
Atkins Quick Quisine Pasta Sides

Condiments
Atkins Quick Quisine Salad Dressings
Atkins Quick Quisine Sauces
Atkins Quick Quisine Sugar Free Pancake Syrup
Atkins Quick Quisine Sugar Free Flavored Syrups

Snacks
Atkins Crunchers Chips

Candy and Frozen Desserts
Atkins Endulge Caramel Nut Chew
Atkins Endulge Chocolate Candy Bars
Atkins Endulge Peanut Butter Cups
Atkins Endulge Wafer Crisp Bars
Atkins Endulge Super Premium Ice Cream Bars
Atkins Endulge Super Premium Ice Cream Cups
Atkins Endulge Super Premium Ice Cream Pints

Index

THERE'S NOTHING TO
EAT ON ATKINS® EXCEPT...

Advantage
bars and shakes

Almond Brownie Bar
Chocolate Peanut
Butter Bar
Café au Lait Shake
Vanilla Shake

Crunchers
snack chips

Original Chips
Nacho Chips
BBQ Chips
Sour Cream & Onion
Chips

Quick Quisine
mixes and pastas

Corn Muffin Mix
Pancake/Waffle Mix
Elbows & Cheese Pasta Side
Fettuccine Alfredo Pasta Side

Supplements
vitamins and minerals

Accel
Basic #3
Dieter's Advantage
Essential Oils

Morning Start
breakfast foods

Cinnamon Bun Bar
Apple Crisp Bar
Banana Nut Harvest Cereal
Crunchy Almond Crisp Cereal

Endulge
chocolate candy

Peanut Butter Cups
Chocolate Mint Wafer
Caramel Nut Chew
Almond Bar

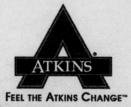

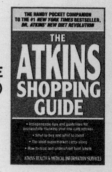

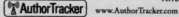